39102000053396
2/20/2007
Berger, Ann
Healing pain :

D1041336

healing
pain

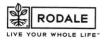

Every day our brands connect with and inspire millions of
people to live a life of the mind, body, spirit — a whole life.

The Innovative,

Breakthrough Plan

to Overcome

Your Physical Pain

& Emotional Suffering

healing
pain

Ann Berger, MSN, MD
and C. B. deSwaan

RODALE

Printed in the United States of America
Rodale Inc. makes every effort to use acid-free ⊗, recycled paper ◉.

Book design by Drew Frantzen

Photo on pages 1 and 93: © Envision/Corbis

Library of Congress Cataloging-in-Publication Data

Berger, Ann (Ann M.)
    Healing pain : the innovative, breakthrough plan to overcome your physical pain and emotional suffering / Ann Berger and C. B. deSwaan.
        p.   cm.
    Includes bibliographical references (p.   ) and index.
    ISBN-13 978–1–59486–012–6 paperback
    ISBN-10 1–59486–012–2 paperback
    1. Chronic pain—Treatment.   2. Chronic pain—Alternative treatment.
I. DeSwaan, Constance.   II. Title.
RB127.B468   2006
616'.0472   2005031077

Distributed to the trade by Holtzbrinck Publishers

2   4   6   8   10   9   7   5   3   1   paperback

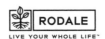

We inspire and enable people to improve their lives and the world around them
For more of our products visit **rodalestore.com** or call 800-848-4735

To my husband, Carl, my children, Stephen and Rebecca,
and my parents, Joseph and Judith Cohen,
whose love and support make my work possible.

To Jane Ann ("Yogiboo") Krauser, who lived her philosophy of hope
and optimism until, at age 43, she lost her long battle with breast
cancer in November 2005. Jane's astonishing spirit, and her
determination to "keep your fork" for life's next offering,
taught me a lot about the real meaning of courage.

contents

acknowledgments

I would like to thank my colleagues—doctors, nurses, counselors, and specialty therapists—who were interviewed for this book and contributed their knowledge and concern.

I want to thank my editor, Amy Super, for her interest in and enthusiasm for this book.

Finally, I want to express my appreciation to the patients and families who continuously teach me about the management of pain and who are the true heroes.

introduction

There's a teacart next to my desk at work, an odd little piece of furniture to keep in a hospital office, but it's precious to me. I keep a formal tea service on the inlaid-wood top tray—exquisite china cups and silver teaspoons that patients have given to me over the years. I've stocked an assortment of teas, sugar, and a variety of flavored honeys and packaged cookies on the bottom shelf. You'll see hats and scarves and a few eye-popping feather boas draped over the teacart's handles, which I give out to patients to wear when we actually sit down and have tea.

The teacart and I have a long history, although its healing uses were not clear until I put it into service at the pain and palliative care department I founded 5 years ago. I *did* know how it made me feel, though. When I was a little girl, I loved tea parties. I would dress my dolls and stuffed animals in my mother's hats and scarves and put on my best dress. When we were all seated at the little table in my room, I'd make an elaborate show of pouring the "tea" and providing all the voices for the lively conversation. This was always fun, but it was much better when I cajoled my parents or another grown-up relative into joining me. My sophisticated mother elevated the conversation, making us both grand ladies at high tea. My father gamely pinched hold of the handle of one of my tiny teacups and told funny stories. I always cherished the memories of these playtimes.

All through medical school, those tea parties summed up in one image an aspect of childhood I wish were more present in my adult life: unconditional love along with an uncensored expression of the joy any one person can have for another—whether it is family or friends for each other, or doctors for patients, or patients for doctors! When I had just graduated from medical school, I spotted what would be "my teacart" in an odd-lots store where my husband and I were buying our moving supplies. The store was in one of the worst neighborhoods of Toledo, and the merchandise for sale was a jumble of yard-sale junk and household necessities. In the middle of this chaos, the teacart stood out like a diamond in a coal bin. As we circled around, picking up this and that, I kept bringing us back to the teacart. Although the $150 price was a fortune for two practical young people just out of graduate school, I couldn't get it off my mind. In the end, Carl and I decided it would be my reward for all my hard work at school. And anyway, who knew? We were moving to Connecticut a week from then, and we thought our life there might be one where a teacart would be *de rigeur.*

As it turned out, we didn't have a tea-party kind of life. We had children and careers instead. The teacart accompanied us to my residency in West Hartford, to my graduate fellowship at Yale, and to Camden, New Jersey, where I set up a pain and palliative care service at the hospital there. After 14 years of wandering with us, the teacart had never been used.

One day I was inspired to talk about it with one of the nurses on my team in Camden. I told Donna that I'd thought of a new use for this neglected beauty—sharing it with patients. After all, I insisted, who wouldn't get a kick out of the Mad Hatter aspect of taking high tea in the middle of the oncology ward? Donna was enthusiastic, but I never got around to bringing in the cart.

When I got the job I have now in Bethesda, Maryland, Donna agreed to make the move and work with me, and we agreed we'd try teacart therapy. At the surprise good-bye party my staff threw for me, attended by 150 of my former patients who had successfully learned how to manage their pain, I was given gifts of tea services, teas, and some of the silly headgear. In one afternoon, my teacart went from being a useless indulgence to a meaningful representation of successful healings. I knew I would be proud to use it at my new job.

And so I did. On the day I decided to debut the teacart, it made an awful racket as I rolled it down the hallway. It hadn't been pushed in 14 years, and every one of the wheels rolled along the floor with a rusty-sounding squeak. My team and I must have left quite an impression as we rattled down the hall to the intensive care unit looking like carnival runaways. There I was, the respected department head, draped in a magenta feather boa, while the rest of my team dressed in floppy hats or brightly colored scarves. People plastered themselves up against the hallway walls as we passed.

We rounded the corner to a room in the oncology ward and came upon a doctor touching his patient gingerly with gloved hands. When he saw the clown posse I was leading, his eyes got huge, and he backed away from the patient and from us. From the look on his face, I thought I'd finally gone too far. Disturbing another doctor's examination was a huge violation of protocol. Our silly outfits probably sealed the breach. Nevertheless, I spoke up confidently.

"Sorry to interrupt you!" I said. "We can come back later."

"Oh, no, no, no, no," the doctor said, taking off his gloves as he backed toward the door. He looked at his patient, who was just beaming. "It's okay. I'll come back," he added.

"You know, I'm a doctor, too," I called after him as he ran out of the room.

From that moment, the teacart proved to be a huge success with the patients, but it didn't boost my credibility with my peers, who, at best, saw it as harmless. They thought that being dressed in an outlandish outfit and having tea with a group of similarly attired, well-trained professionals did not treat physical pain. Yet in a very roundabout way, I believed it spoke to a basic aspect of the healing process.

Something important happens when people connect by humor or by ritual or by unorthodox healing methods. The teacart ritual embodies all these, wherein the doctor, for a moment, discards her need to be the authority figure, and the patient gets to drop her role as the sufferer or the obedient patient. With those two roles put to the side for the duration of the tea taking, doctor and patient are open to each other. For a few minutes, the person focusing on curing an illness and the person seeking a cure are hoisting a cup socially to acknowledge the power of a common goal—to improve the quality of the patient's life. I could feel the brief but intimate connections, and they were powerful.

At last, I felt as if I'd achieved my ambition of re-creating the feeling—in its new form—that I'd gotten when my parents perched on the tiny chairs at my childhood tea table.

A few months after the teacart's debut, I was asked to give "grand rounds," a seminar attended by colleagues during which a doctor explains her research and findings. Grand rounds led by other doctors usually featured their slides of tumors, organs, or cells affected by innovative treatments and a talk augmented with graphs and charts that showed clinical results. In all the grand rounds I'd had the pleasure to attend, I'd never seen a picture of a human being, never mind one smiling.

My team's results can't be plotted on a graph. And the subject of my talk—humanism in medicine and the spiritual concerns of the ill and those in pain—could best be illustrated by photographs of my patients. During the question-and-answer period, one of the top administrators raised his hand and said, "Ann, tell them about your teacart!" I summed up my quest to promote healing by breaking through old traditional doctor-patient barriers, beginning with the teacart. I was met with some agreement, but mostly doubt. One doctor took me aside after my presentation and cautioned: "If you continue on like this, you won't be successful here."

I knew what he was telling me: that being a doctor who lowered her guard and related to patients as equals was threatening to the administration. He was warning me to follow old rules, but I held firm with my approach. The teacart helped me get in touch with patients, and it helped patients stay in touch with the joys in life. I persisted, and I stocked my cart. My colleagues persisted in their doubt, until they finally saw results. Patients really did respond to the intimacy of the "tea party." Ultimately, I was accepted.

Now, when I wheel the well-oiled teacart onto the ward, all examinations stop. Doctors don the silly hats and take a moment out of their jam-packed day to hoist a cup of tea that celebrates their mutual humanity. Doctors are far from being fools. They don't do something antithetical to their training just out of the goodness of their hearts. They do it because, as silly as it sounds and as irrelevant as it seems, the tea party connection works. Healing is enhanced!

Take Tea with Me

I want to start off this book by assuring you that I believe you: Your pain is whatever you say it is and is as bad as you describe it. In fact, in more than 20 years of treating thousands of patients with chronic pain, I've learned that pain is not only as bad as my patients say, it is probably worse. No matter your prognosis, the book you hold in your hands offers you many new chances to heal yourself. The process begins by deciding to step over a few boundaries and, with your doctor's knowledge, expand your healing experiences.

This book contains much of my expertise as a pain management practitioner. But without you, my knowledge cannot make a difference. I hope you will read what these self-help techniques can do to alleviate your pain, and then try them. I fully believe in patient participation rather than patient passivity, and I ask you to give these methods a chance. In other words, I'm asking you to take tea with me.

How This Book Is Set Up to Help You

I've divided the book into two sections, each with a different purpose. In Part 1, I examine what you may be going through physically and emotionally, related to your pain condition. This includes what pain does to you, both physically and psychologically, and how it affects your relationships.

In Part 2, I've included chapters that describe what you can do now to help yourself. This is where *your* efforts enter into your healing process. What you do for yourself truly matters! For example, you'll see why spirituality and deep inner connections help end your sense of feeling like a victim and why being more spiritual fosters healing. You'll learn the importance of improving your optimistic attitude and allowing joy into your life. If you've ever wondered (or worried) about what drugs and surgery can or cannot do for you, I provide the answers to your questions in the chapters on medication and medical procedures. You'll see how some complementary therapies can help relieve pain and what you should know about them. There's a chapter on what the people who care about you should know, and finally, I show you how to create an individualized treatment plan you can follow to make a real difference.

Not every modality will help everyone. But I know that at least one or more of the methods I suggest in this book work for *everyone*—no matter what hurts. Please try some of these ideas and take a step closer to being pain free.

PART 1

understanding pain

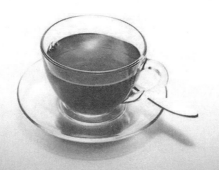

CHAPTER 1

Where Does It Hurt?

The Anatomy of Pain

What is the reason for pain—why do we feel it, how do we feel it, and why does it or doesn't it go away?

I deal with these basic questions every day, treating people whose lives have been overturned by pain. Some are people whose agony is so overwhelming that they can think of little else, and they can do even less. Others are in emotional pain because few people—not the doctors, not their families or friends—believe them when they describe how much they're hurting. It often sounds like this.

- "Some days, my neck feels like it's wrapped in barbed wire, and I can't do a thing or care for my kids."

- "When a migraine hits, I may want to lie in a dark room with ice packs on my forehead, but I get to work managing a busy mall shop and try to pass for normal."

- "I broke my leg skiing, and it's never been the same. Sometimes, the pain in my knee is literally toe curling."

Sound familiar?

Whether we're talking about extreme pain, chronic pain, mild pain, or the degree to which you tolerate pain, one thing is certain: Your response to pain is always unique because pain is supremely subjective. Two people may be able to agree with each other about what a headache generally feels like and that childbirth causes more physical distress than a routine internal examination. They may not, however, agree about exactly which sensations and what degree of intensity constitutes acute pain or an odd and persistent ache.

Agreement or disagreement about "how bad the pain is" is a mystery—to you and to medical professionals. Two people with the identical physical disorder, like a herniated disk or migraines or endometriosis or even cancer, can deal with it in radically different ways: One pops painkillers, while the other takes the stairs two at a time or, like the mall shop manager quoted earlier, fakes her way through the day pretending she is perfectly fine.

What's pain all about?

Understanding How to Heal Yourself

No matter what your prognosis, you can take this chance to heal by being willing to heal yourself. The process begins by assessing your overall health in a different way.

Here's what I mean: In current medical practice, a patient may come in to the hospital complaining of heart palpitations and shortness of breath and saying that she recently has lost a lot of weight. Her doctor orders a million-dollar workup: blood tests, x-rays, a CAT scan, and a biopsy. If he finds, for example, lung cancer, the approach is to attack the disease and destroy it. The patient gets chemotherapy, radiation, and perhaps surgery. The cancer goes into remission, but the patient is still in pain, and she wants relief.

"You shouldn't be having this pain," the doctor chides in disbelief. "I've given you a dozen tests, and there's nothing wrong with you now." Another doctor examines her and offers the same diagnosis: "Take it easy. The pain is all in your head." Not comforting or helpful. The problem: Nobody is looking at the *person* with lung cancer: Who *is* this woman; what does she feel and think about her disease? More, how has her pain or illness affected her life in every aspect— her friendships, family, sexuality, interests, and ability to get around? Has pain altered in any way the connection to her spirituality?

The physical stimulus of pain is only part of what you feel. Total pain can be magnified as much as 100 percent by those other key factors in your life, such as relationships, losses you have not grieved over, work, and financial status. My experience and beliefs prove that unless we treat these factors, thereby treating the whole person and not just the disease, suffering will not abate.

Pain, then, is not just that isolated discomfort, distress, or agony. It has a profile and a personality. My mission in this book is to reveal every aspect of your pain to you. I'll guide you through the same process we would use if you were one of my patients. Yes, we first want to identify the pain and try some things that will lessen its impact on your life. We also want to celebrate your humanity and your individuality and define the legacy you will leave to the world by the courageous way you remain a strong, caring, and loving person despite the circumstances of your condition or illness.

Although pain sounds like a sad and ponderous subject for a book, as you read through, you'll find that my methods make sense in helping you clarify how and why you feel what you do. I hope that through the process, you'll be inspired and motivated to lighten your load by treating pain through the senses, reawakening to what gives you pleasure and joy.

My unique approach to deconstructing the causes of pain and suffering works for anyone with chronic pain—and there are millions of you out there. Statistics reveal that an estimated 70 million Americans endure chronic nonmalignant pain, a problem that experts estimate affects the lives of 20 to 30 percent of the population. Forty percent of Americans get chronic headaches, more than half of us endure significant back pain, and 43 percent are inconvenienced by arthritis and a host of other less common but very painful diseases. Generally, pain is a problem that is not culturally acceptable to reveal, even though some estimates say it has an impact of more than $100 billion a year on the economy. More than 70 percent of us don't want to call the doctor when pain strikes, and almost half of us refuse to take medication until the pain gets really bad.

A *Newsweek* cover story on back pain reported that pain may be pain, but Americans, "especially baby boomers, want a quick fix."

One result is that many people seek a solution in spinal-fusion surgery, the most costly (about $34,000 a pop) and invasive form of therapy, which has spiked dramatically—up 77 percent in the United States between 1996 and 2001. But many procedures, like spinal fusion, don't always totally relieve the pain.

The subject of pain is complicated, so we need to explore its many aspects. Awareness of the different kinds of pain can only help you get a better fix on your own pain cycles and pain triggers. This includes learning how to record them so that you can better discuss them with a doctor.

I know that many of you have good reasons to pick up this book, which offers promise and solutions, especially to those of you who have been dismissed by your doctors and doubted by those you love. So let's begin with hope and let in the humor on this journey of exploration, which, if done properly, will change your life and the lives of those around you.

Why You Feel the Pain You Do

When patients ask me for a definition of pain and where it comes from, my first response is to say that it is the body's sensory network signaling you that something is wrong. The human body was created with pain receptors. Without them, you could not survive. It is as obvious as that: Pain can be a sensory response to actual tissue damage or arise from psychological or spiritual issues. Then again, you don't always see tissue damage with chronic pain.

If I could say that pain has any life-enhancing or life-changing benefits, it's that pain signals protect the body from greater hurt. Think about when you lean against a very hot object with any body part: Nerve endings in your skin react almost instantaneously to produce a reflex action. In a split second, you move away from the thing that could burn you badly. Pain receptors also alert you when internal organs malfunction—kidneys throb, a throat burns, a uterus cramps. The sensation you feel (which you would describe as pain) travels through a complex interactive system in your body. If there is damage to an internal organ, say because of a stomach ulcer, or if you get a black eye or pull your shoulder in a tennis game, nerves start firing.

That pain message from your stomach or eye or shoulder is conveyed along a nerve to the spinal cord, which then shoots it to the part of the brain programmed for that particular sensation. This area of the brain interprets the message, so you can perceive it in a number of ways, including pain, heat, cold, or other sensations. If nerve endings near the source of the pain are not working, then you won't feel the pain. This is why people whose nerves have degenerated from certain diseases or conditions can suffer considerable injuries without noticing. However, some neural damage can have the opposite effect and result in intensified pain, as with some people with herpes simplex. There, damaged neurons send out *more* pain sensations to the brain.

Many types of neurons with different functions are part of this complex system. Pain nerve endings, called nociceptors, are varied and programmed to respond to heat, cold, and physical sensations from objects that are sharp, dull, or somewhere in between. But the physical sensation of pain—a stimulus to the traumatized area and then to the nerve endings—is only one element of what you may be feeling. Pain also exists in the context of how you perceive your life and how you manage the pain.

Not surprisingly, pain can be amplified by the quality of intimate relationships, satisfaction with your life's work, and your spiritual concerns. Unresolved traumas and guilt, losses that have not been grieved over, and troubled relationships act as mirrors for pain. How you live and think reflects back on you and gives you an accurate picture. So, to treat pain, we have to look at all its aspects.

Everyone knows what most pain is like, but it can be difficult for a person who has never experienced wrenching, disabling pain to comprehend another's misery. A knowledge of biology, a degree from a medical school, or even compassion for another human being cannot always guarantee understanding or correct treatment. That's because there's something called suffering.

There's a significant difference between pain and suffering, even though most people consider them essentially the same thing.

Pain is the discomfort caused by a physical malady.

Suffering reflects the degree to which people are capable of enduring their pain and involves psychological-social-spiritual issues and questions like "Why me?" Suffering, therefore, also reflects a patient's attitudes about the psychosocial-spiritual elements of life, such as a connection to a higher being or the greatness of the universe, as well as issues of loss and a belief that one's life has meaning and purpose.

Total pain is physical pain plus suffering. Because of this irrevocable connection between mind and body, healing pain must involve both. What you think and feel about pain makes the difference. The stories you tell yourself and others about pain actually organize and make sense of what you're going through.

Suffering cannot just be relieved with a medication like an antidepressant, because there is no medication for suffering. To help relieve suffering, one must consider and include personal relationships, spiritual care, recreation therapy, bodywork (such as massage or Reiki), and other therapies, which are all covered in later chapters.

Pain, Endorphins, and the Hormone Factor

While it's true that pain itself can suppress the immune system and elevate blood pressure, the body can also produce miraculous healing and its own painkillers called endorphins. These are "feel good" hormones. Normally, it takes a physical or emotional trauma and a fight-or-flight response to make the body pump them out.

When you hear about people at accident sites who perform physical actions that should have been impossible because of their injuries and severe pain, their feats are due in part to endorphins. After a time, fewer endorphins are produced to counter the same amount of pain. The body cannot remain in that fight-or-flight mode for long without exhaustion. Chronic pain does not evoke this kind of endorphin response. In fact, there are a few studies that suggest chronic pain patients may produce fewer endorphins.

Endorphins not only change the way you feel about pain, they change the way you feel about the pain you feel—just as drugs like opiates do. Because of endorphins, pain is much less intense, and you

WHAT PAIN CAN DO

Pain takes its toll on personal lives, working lives, and inner lives. The latest statistics from the American Pain Foundation show that 75 million people experience chronic pain related to a nonmalignant condition or a malignancy.

- In terms of having unrelieved pain, 40 percent of sufferers report that their pain is "out of control." In the general public, 70 percent avoid calling a doctor when in pain, 46 percent avoid medication until the pain "gets bad" and 35 percent avoid medication until the pain is "unbearable."

- Chronic pain sufferers tend to be undertreated because diagnostic tests often fail to identify the cause of the problem. Therefore, it's not unusual for them to consult one specialist after another—and some people may even see up to 100 doctors.

- Findings of a recent study done during a specific 2-week period showed that 13 percent of the total workforce lost productivity due to common pain conditions: Headache was the most common pain, followed by back pain, then arthritis pain and other musculoskeletal pain.

- Lost productive time among normally active workers costs an estimated $61.2 to $100 billion a year. The majority of lost productive time (76.6 percent) is shown to be because of either reduced performance at work or work not done.

- For reasons no one can yet explain, women appear to be more susceptible to pain than men. Women are more inclined to describe their pain in terms of feelings and are more likely to hear doctors dismiss their problems as being "psychological."

can even feel detached from it. At its most basic level, the "ouch" of pain is transformed to the "ooh" of relief. Pain may still be talking to you, but it is no longer howling for your attention. However, you do not get used to the pain if you have a chronic pain condition and pain becomes harder to endure.

How Stress Affects Your Pain

A patient with serious migraines told me she'd left work and gotten stuck in the subway on the way home. After a few minutes underground, with the lights off, Loretta began to feel "ill all over," and her head felt like it had been "shot through with glass." She tried to calm herself, since there was nothing she could do to get the train up and running or walk out of there.

What happened to Loretta also happens to you, depending on circumstances. Your sympathetic nervous system causes your body to respond to danger, adversity, stress, anger, and even ecstasy by increasing your heart rate, raising your blood pressure, boosting the air exchange volume of your lungs, and increasing blood flow to your muscles. This part of your nervous system prepares you for action and is regulated by four glands, the hypothalamus, the pituitary, and the adrenals, sometimes referred to as the (HPA) axis.

During periods of extreme emotional stress, the sympathetic nervous system is activated again and again. If the stress continues long enough, the body cannot release all the accumulated tension and retains some of it. That leftover tension mounts until it causes pain. Pain causes more stress, which causes more pain. Unless stress is relieved, an ever-increasing spiral develops, and you're caught right in the middle.

Pain and Gender

Interestingly, new research on pain shows that women tend to report more severe and persistent pain than do men. We all know that people have different thresholds for pain. But thanks to today's sophisticated brain-imaging equipment, scientists can now see those variations in action by using positron emission tomography (PET) scans. One such study was led by Jon-Kar Zubieta, MD, PhD, at the University of Michigan in Ann Arbor. He and his team did tests to see if our painkilling systems can behave in radically different ways, depending on circumstance, gender, and heredity. Dr. Zubieta's team found that women's painkilling systems were, in fact, much more active on estrogen and women's response to pain less pronounced.

While their painkilling systems are more active, women are still more likely to seek medical attention if they need it. It is more culturally acceptable for women to see a doctor for pain relief. In my experience, men are more likely to put off medical attention for pain unless it is extreme or even incapacitating.

Another study showed that gender, and even hair color, can cause different reactions to treatment. Women have been found to be more responsive to a class of painkillers called kappa opioids than are men. Jeffrey Mogil, PhD, a pain expert at McGill University in Montreal, recently reported that he'd found a culprit, a gene called melanocortin-1, which somehow increases sensitivity to kappa opioids and is also responsible for red hair and fair skin. In a pain test, men and women of all hair colors felt similar distress, but female redheads did a lot better on the drugs! "The data suggest that males and females use different circuitry to modulate pain," says Dr. Mogil.

The isolation of genes linked to pain brings a vast new understanding of how individual responses to pain are triggered. Dr. Zubieta's team also discovered that a small variation in a gene called COMT, which helps regulate the brain chemicals dopamine and noradrenaline, separates the sensitive from the steadfast when it comes to putting up with pain.

The discovery of pain-related genes opens up a new frontier for drug development. Biotech companies are eager to exploit such discoveries, the goal of which is to develop new drugs that attack specific chemical processes in pain instead of launching a full-body attack. One day, pain treatments will vary by individual. Your doctor will be able to examine your genetic makeup and then prescribe a drug that will work specifically for you.

Types of Pain

It's clear that pain is understood by anyone and that everyone feels it a bit differently. Overall, pain is an unpleasant sensation that occurs in varying degrees of severity and is a consequence of a number of processes. In order to manage pain, doctors discern its intensity and frequency and the circumstance from which it springs.

Pain is typically categorized into two broad areas: *acute* and *chronic*. Acute pain is easier to diagnose and treat than chronic pain. It usually occurs after an injury, and people in this state look like they're in pain. This type of pain usually disappears when the injury heals. If you break your nose in a fall or cut yourself in your workroom, you probably feel the pain pulsing like a silent alarm throughout your body. With acute pain, your heart rate, respiratory rate, fight-or-flight response, and sweating increase. While acute pain is severe, the good news is that it lasts a relatively short time.

Chronic pain is a lot more complex.

A Closer Look at Chronic Pain

An article on chronic pain in the *Journal of the American Medical Association* noted that chronic pain is expensive, mainly because of the resulting disability and absence from work. In recent studies, researchers say, "more attention has been paid to the impact of chronic pain on daily living." And what an impact it has.

What *is* chronic pain? A typical definition says that chronic pain is not one thing, but a condition that varies depending on the person. The variables include where the pain is, what its cause is, and how an injury heals. In some cases, the pain is simply inexplicable. However, one description is consistently applicable: All chronic pain is long-term pain that persists even after healing has occurred or when the condition that's causing the pain does not go away. This is pain beyond what doctors expect to see from a condition or injury that does clear up.

Some women with endometriosis have worse symptoms during their cycles, while others begin feeling pain a week before that. When these women describe their pain as chronic, it's because they're uncomfortable for at least 2 weeks of the month. People who get bad migraines usually experience them intermittently rather than every day. So in that way, you may perceive your migraines as not actually being chronic, but recurring. I also get migraines once a month, but I don't consider the condition chronic. Healing starts here! Chronic pain cannot have power over your thinking when you at least partly define it as something you will not allow to affect how you function.

Unlike people in the throes of acute pain, patients with chronic pain often do not appear to be in pain—but indeed they are! Research done with chronic pain sufferers shows that some exhibit greater brain activity than healthy people when subjected to pain. This may be why they experience pain more severely. Yet, they've gotten good at "getting through" and soldiering on. Rather than seeing an elevated change in vital signs, like increased heart rate, one usually sees vegetative signs, and, not to be dismissed, such a person may appear depressed.

People with chronic pain tell me that they have sleep disturbances, decreased libido, anhedonia (an inability to feel pleasure), constipation, lethargy, and personality change; lose their appetites; and sometimes are preoccupied with their bodies. These are all classic symptoms of chronic pain. But why the pain? Often, it's due to a disease, while at other times, it's the treatment of the disease that produces the pain. When a person has any type of surgery, they can be left with a long-term pain problem secondary to scarring, or even permanent nerve damage.

Chronic or persistent pain may range from mild to severe, and it is present to some degree for long periods of time. Some people with chronic pain that is controlled by medication can have "breakthrough pain," which occurs when the medication does not work and moderate to severe pain breaks through or is felt for a short time. This can occur several times a day, even when the proper dose of medicine is given.

In treating chronic pain, it's important to understand the different potential types and mechanisms of pain.

Referred pain is felt some distance from where the pain actually originates. In other words, the site of the pain is not necessarily the source. Osteoarthritis of the hip, for example, causes pain to be experienced in the knee. In acupuncture, a form of Chinese medicine, kidney problems can be indicated by pain in the knees.

Phantom pain occurs when you have had a limb, breast, or other body part removed by surgery. People describe the pain or unpleasant sensations as if they were coming from the absent body part, but phantom pain is real and not in patients' minds.

Somatic pain is caused by activation of a pain receptor. Remember, pain nerve endings, called nociceptors, are programmed to respond to various stimuli, such as heat, cold, and other physical sensations. The characteristics of the pain are very well localized aching, throbbing, and a gnawing feeling. Examples include joint and bone pain. This type of pain is generally very responsive to nonsteroidal anti-inflammatory drugs (NSAIDs) like aspirin, and when they are no longer helpful, one can use opiate medications to treat this type of pain.

Visceral pain is also caused by activation of a pain receptor. The patient often feels achy, vaguely localized pain. It commonly originates in the abdomen or the chest, it does not feel as if it is limited to only one area. A good example of visceral pain is chest pain due to a heart attack. In this case, the pain occurs in the chest, but it can go up the neck and down the arm, too. This type of pain is a little more difficult to treat, but it can respond to opiates and adjuvant medications.

Neuropathic pain is caused by destruction of a nerve in either the peripheral or central nervous system. Neuropathy can be best thought of as a seizure of a nerve. People often describe a severe, sharp, shooting, or stabbing pain or a burning, numb, or tingling sensation.

Myofascial pain is muscle pain that occurs in conjunction with other pains. The trigger point is a localized, highly irritable spot in a taut band of skeletal muscle. Palpation of these trigger points will alter the pain, causing it to increase or radiate. You may feel as if you are having a muscle spasm.

How You Feel Pain: Communicating about Pain So Others Understand

Each of us has a pain threshold, which is a combination of psychological and neurological factors. At one extreme, stoics and mind-control practitioners may choose to feel no pain—some can even stanch the flow of blood from a wound by use of willpower alone. At the other extreme, there are people who suffer and whom nobody believes—and who are unfairly labeled hypochondriacs. Regardless, what matters most is that you describe your pain accurately enough in all its varying degrees and severity so that others can understand and help relieve it.

The ability to communicate a private sense of pain to a medical professional gives you a better chance to get the most effective medical help. But what happens when communication is thwarted by a physician who invalidates a patient's report of pain?

WORDS THAT DESCRIBE HOW YOUR PAIN REALLY FEELS

Since describing pain to your doctor is important, you can acquaint yourself with the language to understand it better. Pain can be:

- Pulsing, throbbing, pounding, shooting, prickling, stabbing, lancing, electric, sharp, pinching, gnawing, cramping, crushing, tugging, wrenching, hot, killing, blinding, intense, unbearable, spreading, radiating, piercing, tearing, agonizing

- Tingling, itching, smarting, stinging, dull, sore, aching, heavy, tender, taut, tiring, exhausting, sickening, suffocating, frightful, annoying, troublesome, tight, rigid, numbing, drawing, squeezing, cold, icy, nagging

---

For women whose doctors have told them repeatedly that the pain they feel does not exist, emotional turmoil may become as much a symptom of a condition like endometriosis as the actual physical disability. As a treatment, some doctors may prescribe Valium or other tranquilizers, not realizing that these drugs don't help the pain. Generally, when pain persists, another doctor is consulted. Should he or she concur with the first, this doctor may simply prescribe stronger tranquilizers, and a woman's illness becomes doubly wearing. Her self-doubt begins to grow as her pain increases in severity. The questions such a woman asks herself remain unanswered: "How am I creating such horrible pain? How can I stop doing this to myself?"

Clearly, this situation is emotionally wrenching. Rather than being able to follow their own inner voices, which tell them that this pain means something, many of these women are made to feel defeated, somehow responsible—and guilty—until the disease becomes so advanced and so serious that even a minimally experienced physician is able to diagnose it. Cathy's experience tells such a story.

Cathy came to see me after she heard me lecture at a women's interest group that focused on contemporary health issues and pain management. She told me her recent medical history, and I was shocked at how, in her case, doctors seemed to treat the symptoms rather than the source of pain. This is what happened, as Cathy told it.

"I'm 38 years old and for most of my life, I've been healthy. I got married 13 years ago, I had twins the first year we were married, and my husband and I decided not to have any more children. About a year ago, life changed for me. One morning, I awakened with a burning pain and a feeling of vaginal pressure." She went to a gynecologist, who diagnosed vaginitis. To be certain, the doctor took a few cultures, which came up negative. Cathy was still in pain, but the doctor had no solutions for her, and in fact, she reported, things got worse.

Cathy then went to another doctor, who tested her for chlamydia, a venereal disease. That test came out negative, too. Meanwhile, she was feeling worse and dealing with rectal pain as well.

She found a third gynecologist, who played around with pills and other medication for a fungal infection that he next decided Cathy had. She was in horrible pain—in addition to having menstrual cramps—so he did a sonogram. It showed nothing.

Five months passed, and the pain began to shift, this time clearly to Cathy's urinary tract. She went to a urologist, who said she had stenosis—a narrowing of the urethra. He dilated her urethra, a procedure that was a nightmare for her and caused her tremendous pain. He also gave Cathy a topical cream to apply, which didn't help. "Worse," she added, "along with everything else, intercourse was painful."

In all, Cathy saw four doctors, and she felt none had taken her pain seriously. Finally, after a year had passed, a fifth doctor did a laparoscopy and found why Cathy was in pain—she had endometriosis. She said, "I feel such frustration over this, since I know I'd have been in much better shape if the first doctor had taken me seriously and had considered endometriosis as a possible problem."

What happened to Cathy sometimes occurs when doctors focus on the most obvious sites of pain. We know that vaginal pain need not always indicate a localized infection, just as pain during urination need not implicate only the urinary tract. Cathy also got caught seeing doctors who failed to diagnose endometriosis early on, which makes a difference for any woman who has the malady. Armed with knowledge and the right treatment, a woman with endometriosis can head toward a normal, joyous, fulfilling life with bearable and manageable pain.

Where Does It Hurt?

In providing all the scientific explanations about pain, I hope to help you understand what pain is, but this is just the beginning. What really matters is that you understand your own pain so you can do as much as possible to relieve it. To do this, you need to learn how to connect with what's happening in your body and mind—listen to yourself, so to speak, and really hear what's going on—an ability that's not half as easy as it sounds.

In a world crowded with stimulation, distortions, and demands, we've almost lost the faculty to tune in to ourselves accurately.

Consider all the external distractions in your day; you've probably heard yourself say, "I can't hear myself think!" To really listen, you have to put aside your more superficial thoughts and sit still long enough to hear how you really feel.

How *do* you feel? It seems like a simple question. It's something we ask each other all the time without really expecting a truthful reply. You bump into a friend at the mall and ask, "How are you?" If that friend answered, "I've got a pain in my leg. I just had a fight with my son, and I'm very agitated. Things are tough at work, and I'm worried about getting fired. The economy is so bad. But it's a beautiful day, and I'm distracting myself with shopping," you wouldn't know how to respond. We want to hear "Fine." We want to say "Fine." In our heart of hearts, that's what we hope for, after all, and it's the message we want to spread to the world.

What's so remarkable about the exchange above isn't just the shock of the friend's candor. Most people don't know how they feel. In fact, when asked to answer that question truthfully, most wouldn't know where to start. The goal of this chapter is to show you how to make a candid self-assessment, an important first step in healing.

When I meet a patient for the first time, I take a deep breath before I enter the room to clear my head of all that may be bothering me so I can focus completely on the person who sits before me. I have already reviewed the patient's file to familiarize myself with the medical facts of the case, but I put aside that knowledge before we meet so I can open myself to the person. I hope to show you how to pay this kind of attention to yourself. As with my ritual, I'd like you to start by taking time to breathe.

The Connection between Healing Breath and Pain

I know that sounds a bit silly. We were born knowing how to breathe. We couldn't live without the oxygen that feeds our systems, but in times of stress or when our bodies are shut down because of illness, our breathing frequently becomes shallow and halting—a sign to ourselves and the world that we don't think we deserve to take up so much oxygen. We take in just enough to keep everything operating, but we refuse to draw in the deep, slow, centering breath that clears away all the distractions and allows us to really experience our bodies and the world around us. This is the kind of breath I want you to take while we figure out exactly where it hurts.

Notice your breathing right now. How would you describe it? Does your breath go in and out in short little puffs? Or does it stutter with momentary gaps between inhale and exhale? The goal of this initial exercise is to teach you to take long, slow, steady breaths, a simple and easily accessible form of stress reduction. Read the following paragraph all the way through and then try the exercise.

Sit comfortably with your hands relaxed on your lap and close your eyes. Notice your breathing as it is right now. Pause after the exhale and start slowly on your next inhale. Try to lengthen the inhale by just a few seconds. Pause and try to make the exhale the same length as the inhale. Try again. As you continue with this exercise for 5 to 10 breaths, try to make each breath a little bit longer on each side of the pause. Have you ever watched babies breathe? Their whole abdomen fills with the air they take in. Eventually, as you focus on the breath, yours will, too. Your goal is to learn to breathe like a baby.

Long, deep breaths cleanse me of stress and root my attention in my body. By centering my attention at my core—the heart and the lungs—I feel alert, with all my senses open yet beautifully still. The stillness creates the perfect atmosphere for me to listen to what patients have to tell me. I want to be calm and free of judgment so that I can absorb as much as possible about my patients' conditions. Every gesture and word choice expresses something, and only by being still and open can I understand the true nature of my patients' pain so we can start seeking the most effective treatments.

I regret I can't be there with you as you explore the story of your pain, but my hope is that I can describe my method well enough that you can find these answers for yourself. Understanding your pain—its history, cycle, and origins—is the fundamental first step in healing. I think of that wise assessment from the 12-step movement: Once I accept myself as I am, then I can better understand what's right about me and what I need to change.

This moment is as good a place to start as any. Where are you sitting as you read this? Are you hunched over a hurried lunch? Sitting propped up in bed? In a favorite chair? Take a few more deep breaths. How do you feel? Consider this question in a different fashion: What is the order of importance you give sensations? Some people start with the physical pain first. Others may be more aware of their emotions. All of this is important to the total picture of your pain, as every sensation you feel helps you to better understand your unique situation at this moment.

To help you better describe this large territory, I'm including the many questions I would ask if we were seated together and about to begin your treatment plan.

How You Feel Right Now

Answer as many of these questions as you can in the first reading, then go back and answer the remaining questions. The more you know about yourself, the better and faster you will heal.

• How long have you been in pain?

_____

_____

• Where is it most painful right now?

_____

_____

• Has this changed from your initial complaint?

_____

_____

- How would you describe this pain? (See "Words That Describe How Your Pain Really Feels" on page 15 for help describing your pain.)

_____

_____

- Right now, where would you rate the pain on a scale of 0 to 10 (with 10 being the worst pain)?

_____

_____

- What has the pain been like in the last 24 hours?

_____

_____

- What has it been like in the last week?

_____

_____

- What aggravates the pain? Moving? Standing? Sitting?

_____

_____

- What alleviates it? Heat? Cold? Massage?

_____

_____

- What medications are you on? Include herbal, over-the-counter, and doctor-prescribed medicines.

_____

_____

- Do you experience any side effects from these medicines?

_____

_____

- Is there any aspect of your pain that is not addressed by these medications?

_____

_____

- Since your illness began, have you had:

☐ Weight change

☐ Change in eating habits, including reduction in appetite

☐ Fatigue

☐ Diarrhea

☐ Nausea/vomiting

☐ Indigestion

☐ Constipation

☐ Anemia

☐ Skin problems

☐ Heart rhythm irregularities

☐ Edema (swelling)

☐ Headaches

☐ Sleep difficulties like insomnia or night sweats

☐ Sensory disturbances, such as changed vision, balance, hearing, taste, or touch

☐ Motor coordination problems

☐ Concentration difficulties or memory lapses

☐ Alertness problems or confusion

☐ Urinary or sexual difficulties

• Have you experienced any side effects from other therapeutic treatments?

_____

_____

• What is your smoking history? If you smoke now, how many packs a day/week?

_____

_____

• Do you drink? How many drinks a week, on average?

_____

_____

• Do you take illicit drugs? If so, which kinds and how often?

_____

_____

Your Support System

Chapter 3 goes into this subject in depth, but please answer these questions as best you can now.

• Do you feel loved?

_____

_____

• Are you married/divorced/widowed/single? Do you have children? Pets?

_____

_____

• With whom do you live?

_____

_____

• Do you believe you are getting emotional support from your family?

_____

_____

• Do you feel close to your friends?

_____

_____

- Are your friends supportive?

_____

_____

- Do you think you are communicating effectively with your friends and family about your illness?

_____

_____

- Do you feel close to the person who is your main support?

_____

_____

- Do you think this person understands what you are going through?

_____

_____

- Are you satisfied with your sex life?

_____

_____

- Whom do you see regularly?

_____

_____

• On whom can you depend?

_____

_____

• Whom do you trust?

_____

_____

• Who validates your point of view?

_____

_____

• Who seems rushed and distracted when you describe your condition?

_____

_____

• With whom are you fighting?

_____

_____

• Are there some relationships you consider to be a burden?

_____

_____

Your Place in the World

- Are you able to work?

_____

_____

- Do you have financial difficulties?

_____

_____

- Are you able to fulfill your responsibilities at home?

_____

_____

- Have you had to cut back on your activities?

_____

_____

- Do you have trouble doing the things you used to do?

_____

_____

- Do you need help in the normal running of the house?

_____

_____

• Do you have trouble meeting the needs of your family?

_____

_____

• Are you forced to spend time in bed?

_____

_____

YOUR EMOTIONAL STATE

• Have you accepted your illness?

_____

_____

• Are you anxious?

_____

_____

• Are you sad?

_____

_____

• Do you feel lonely?

_____

_____

• Do you worry that your condition will get worse?

_____

_____

• Is your work fulfilling?

_____

_____

• Are you content with the present quality of your life?

_____

_____

• Do you have trouble feeling peace of mind?

_____

_____

• Can you comfort yourself?

_____

_____

• Do you think that whatever happens with your illness, things will be okay?

_____

_____

Your Family History

- Is there a history of depression in your family, treated or untreated?

_____

_____

- If some of your family members have died, what was the cause?

_____

_____

- What kinds of relationships did you have with them?

_____

_____

- Are you estranged from any members of your family?

_____

_____

- Are there episodes with your family that you regret?

_____

_____

- What was your family's coping style? For example, were problems out in the open? Or were problems not talked about, denied, or talked about in hushed tones? Could you easily talk about your needs or wishes? Were your feelings or interests honored and respected, or were they diminished and belittled by parents who needed to exert control over you?

_____

_____

Spiritual Concerns

Chapter 4 goes into this subject in depth, but please answer these questions now.

• Do you consider yourself to be spiritual or religious?

_____

_____

• Do you have spiritual beliefs that have helped you cope with your illness?

_____

_____

• What importance does faith or belief have in your life?

_____

_____

- Have your beliefs influenced how you have taken care of yourself in this illness?

_____

_____

- What role do your beliefs play in regaining your health?

_____

_____

- Are you part of a spiritual or religious community?

_____

_____

- Has illness strengthened your faith?

_____

_____

- Do you worry about dying?

_____

_____

- Do you feel you have a reason for living?

_____

_____

- Do you think your life has been productive?

_____

_____

- Do you have a sense of meaning and purpose?

_____

_____

Beginning to Take Charge of Your Pain

Today, we know that pain should never be ignored. It should be assessed thoroughly, treated aggressively, and, in some cases, managed as a chronic condition. We've learned that when pain is managed, stress is reduced and the body heals faster.

When people with pain work together with their health-care professionals and take an active role in their pain management, they get the best results possible—less pain and more involvement in life. But it must begin with you.

Since you're the only one who knows the degree to which you feel pain, what you tell your doctor or other health-care professional makes a big difference in getting the best care. One of the best ways I know to provide the most accurate information about the pain you're feeling is to keep a daily pain journal, or log. This gives your medical team an idea of changes in your pain over time.

I've put together three different logs that you can use every day—each one asking for different information only you can fill in. The first log allows you to gauge the intensity of your pain and rate it from 0 to 10, with 10 being the worst pain. The second allows you to describe your pain in detail, and the third asks you to track your use of medications and whether they do or don't make you feel better.

To get the most out of these logs:

- Track your pain every day for at least 2 weeks. (There are copies of these logs in the Appendix so you can use the ones here and duplicate the others to track your pain for another 2 weeks or more.)

- Write down as much information as you can think of about your pain.

- Don't hold back on how you're feeling. You have no reason to be embarrassed or afraid to reveal this information to your doctor.

- Fill in all sections of the journal. If you're not able to complete the journal every day, ask someone to help you with the task so that you track your pain for at least 1 week.

DAILY PAIN LEVEL LOG

FIRST WEEK

Pain	Mon.	Tues.	Wed.	Thur.	Fri.	Sat.	Sun.
10							
9							
8							
7							
6							
5							
4							
3							
2							
1							
0							

It doesn't take very long to record the information about how you feel, so promise yourself to faithfully fill in the log every day.

1. Tracking Your Pain Level Day by Day

- In the chart below, make a check mark in the box that corresponds with the day of the week and your specific pain level. For example, if it is Tuesday, and you had moderate to more severe neck pain, you might enter a check mark in the Tuesday column corresponding to number 6 or 7.

- At the end of each day, answer the questions in Step 2, providing specific information about the pain you did or didn't feel that day.

Weeks of _____

SECOND WEEK							
Pain	Mon.	Tues.	Wed.	Thur.	Fri.	Sat.	Sun.
10							
9							
8							
7							
6							
5							
4							
3							
2							
1							
0							

2. Describing Your Pain Day by Day

Write down what did or didn't happen to you because of the pain. You can use the Daily Pain Description Log on page 38. Provide as much information as possible about your pain level by answering these questions.

- How many times did you feel pain? It could be none, once, 10 times, for example, however many times it happened.

- List where you felt pain. Was it, for example, in your neck, back, wrists, abdominal area, or all over your body?

- Did any specific activity start the pain? If so, which activity? Were you, for example, climbing stairs, lifting a child, or doing chores such as laundry, vacuuming, and so on?

- How did the pain interfere with your normal activities, such as sleeping, eating, sexual activity, or working efficiently?

- Every day, note if you avoided, limited, or canceled any activity or social engagement because of pain or changes in how you felt, including working at your job. What changes did you make?

- Did you call your health-care professional between visits because of pain?

So, for example, your entry for Tuesday might read:
"Felt sharp, pulling pain four times in neck. Pain started up driving to work, getting caught in traffic jam, and having to keep turning my head. Slight slowdown at work until late afternoon because of intense, stiffening neck pain and pounding headache. Canceled dinner with my in-laws."

3. Medications, Treatments, and Therapies

The chart on page 40 will help you track how medications, treatments, and therapies do or do not affect your pain. There are six simple questions, and they should take you only a minute or two to answer.

- What is the name of the medication? Did you take it according to your doctor's instructions?

- Did you skip a dose? If so, why?

- Did the medication help relieve your pain?

- Did you still have breakthrough pain even though you took the medication?

- Did you have any side effects after taking the medication?

- Did you do anything to help relieve your pain other than take prescription medication? For example, did you exercise; have physical therapy; take nonprescription drugs, such as ibuprofen or aspirin; use hot or cold packs, get a massage; have acupuncture, Reiki, or other complementary treatments; use relaxation techniques, such as meditation or hypnosis; take a nap; try changing positions, such as lying down and elevating your legs; go for psychological therapy; or do something creative, such as painting, taking a dance class, or doing nonstressful DIY jobs around the house?

For example, on Wednesday, you might write:

"Neck pain woke me up last night so took two aspirin. This morning, pain felt like it was pulling or sharp; took a Percocet to relieve it. Felt better for 4 hours. Headache developed late afternoon, but was bearable. Took another Percocet and felt better. After work, took hot bath, massaged neck."

Never Give Up in Your Fight to Heal Yourself

I'm not going to kid you here. There will still be times when the pain will be overwhelming and days when it will be hard to get out

(continued on page 42)

DAILY PAIN DESCRIPTION LOG

FIRST WEEK

MONDAY	
TUESDAY	
WEDNESDAY	
THURSDAY	
FRIDAY	
SATURDAY	
SUNDAY	

SECOND WEEK

MONDAY	
TUESDAY	
WEDNESDAY	
THURSDAY	
FRIDAY	
SATURDAY	
SUNDAY	

MEDICATION AND TREATMENT LOG

FIRST WEEK

MONDAY	
TUESDAY	
WEDNESDAY	
THURSDAY	
FRIDAY	
SATURDAY	
SUNDAY	

SECOND WEEK

MONDAY	
TUESDAY	
WEDNESDAY	
THURSDAY	
FRIDAY	
SATURDAY	
SUNDAY	

of bed. But the process of healing can also be a lot of fun. Everyone has only one life out of which to get the most. Life is also a journey—you can't change the past, but you can affect the present and the future. You have the gift of knowing this and activating your own motivation to live authentically and take better care of yourself and others.

CHAPTER 2

Why Me?

When You Feel the Pain
You're *Really* Feeling

. . . .

"What if I told you that I've seen nine doctors in the last 3 years and that each one basically told me the same thing in different words, which is: 'There's no reason for the pain in your breast. We took out the tumor, and there are no artifacts from the surgery.' They usually go on to add some advice like 'Take it easy or take antianxiety medication.' When nine specialists tell you that nothing's wrong, but you still feel a pain behind a scar in your breast almost every day, you start having doubts about your mental state!"

—Terri, 38 years old

"I've had knee problems since I was 18 years old, the result of a few football injuries. I've gone through dozens of procedures and two surgeries, which would either help temporarily or not, then I'd be in agony again. I've got a business to run, so I'm at work unless I can't get out of bed. Even then, I'm on the phone all day, half of me on an adrenaline rush, the other half feeling crippled. Name the specialist and I've seen him. Who's got an answer for me?"

—*Tom, 50 years old*

. . . .

Since I treat people whose lives have been altered by pain of one sort or another, I know that physical symptoms are only half of the story. Chronic pain, especially if it's severe, can shift the patterns of how you live your life, affecting your personality. At the most extreme, pain shapes your days—and it's not a long way from that situation to thinking that pain is the subject of your life.

Relieving that pain, though, can be the object of your strength. I can show you how to make this happen for you. The first key is to examine the connection between the physical and psychological aspects of pain.

The Moods of Chronic Pain

Chronic pain is as complex as it is physiologically and psychologically distinct for every one of us. I personally have a high pain threshold and can function pretty well with migraines or back pain— not that I'm not aware of how the disorder makes me feel. I can put it to the side, so to speak, and move along. Others, I know, have different levels of sensitivity and different coping styles, and they are flattened by headaches, endometriosis, carpal tunnel syndrome, arthritis, fibromyalgia, and other such pain-inducing disorders. If I've discovered any one truth in my field, it is that your interpretation of the pain or how you cope with it can make the difference in your healing process. This is what I want to do for you: give you more than hope—give you real and effective solutions you can use and adapt!

When pain takes over, it's very demanding—it's the 900-pound gorilla wound up and ready to spring. Your day is built around the highs of temporary relief when "the beast" is under control and you can function as close to normal as possible. Or, your day may be organized around the lows of distress when you're hurting too much to think about anything else, and you simply shut down. I've treated every level of pain patient.

Many of the people I see have been referred by doctors who aren't trained in pain management, but these doctors have done what they could within their medical specialties. Finally at a loss as to what to do next, colleagues who know of my work will say, "Annie fixes this kind of person. Send him to her!" It's not uncommon for me to begin caring for people who have started to believe they'll never have normal lives again.

The context of pain at this level matters a great deal. When pain cheats you of the familiar interactions you usually take for granted, the situation seems utterly gloomy. Incapacitation can make you less available as a parent, partner, friend, lover, and loyal employee. It's just not a good day when pain makes you back away from relationships, interests, and future goals so you can put all your energy into getting through.

In a less extreme case, you may cope with chronic pain but get no long-term relief from treatments or therapies. Something is missing, and you're not sure what it is or how to talk about it; you're just not feeling better when doctors and your family say you should. More exasperating, though, is fearing that you've "lost it" or that you're "nuts" because you still feel pain even when using the medications or therapies that are supposed to solve the problem.

Is there a way to heal pain? Most definitely.

Life's not about suffering, after all, but about faith—in yourself, in some sort of spiritual connection, and in your ability to create meaningful ties to others and share the creative and even mundane experiences that shape your life. That's not all. Pain need not rule. You also need faith to believe you can be healthy and work toward a balance of body and spirit. Health and happiness almost never spring from suffering and pain.

With faith in your ability to heal yourself, there is one other quality that can help get you through the agony, shock, or changes in your life that result from pain: flexibility. To relieve pain, you have to extend your thinking beyond its usual borders and be willing to try something new. So here, I'm asking you to have faith in my techniques. Give the concepts and suggested therapies I offer in this book a chance, and please do so with an open mind. They can only help.

Putting Pain in Perspective: Tracking the *Why* Behind Your Pain

When I first started out with a specialty in pain, I'd come from an oncology background. I found to my surprise that many pain patients were suffering a lot more than cancer patients who were dying. This troubled me, but as a scientist, I had to examine why.

The onset of chronic pain brings profound psychological changes that fall into a wide range of responses—from disbelief and depression to anger, anxiety, helplessness, hopelessness, and fear. I've found that a lot of people who are depressed have chronic pain, making it tough to determine which came first. In addition, the psychological hot buttons you're dealing with before the pain begins are amplified by physical discomfort, especially if the pain becomes chronic. Beyond this state of affairs, both medical professionals and loved ones may hint that your pain isn't real—a sign that you have a condition to be cured—but rather that you're overdramatizing or imagining either a slight or nonexistent condition. It is incredibly frustrating when you know you're in pain and others don't believe you. This happens more typically with women who complain of, for example, breast pain (as with Terri, whose testimony opens the chapter) or distress from endometriosis.

Treating pain patients requires a more psychologically expansive mind-set for the doctor and for the patient. Medication is often an important part of the healing equation, but real transformation only occurs by treating each patient as a whole person with a soul, not as an embodiment of a disorder.

Let's begin by looking at the first four psychologically related questions that tend to come up when pain becomes chronic.

- Is the pain real, or am I nuts?

- Why am I depressed?

- Why am I feeling stressed?

- Can how I think really make a difference in how I heal?

Is the Pain Real, or Am I Nuts?

When it's pain at a surgery site, as with Terri, or if your problem is migraines, arthritis, an accident-related injury, endometriosis, or even an undiagnosed condition, you know how it feels when pain is your constant companion: You may be stressed, depressed, or frustrated—but determined to beat it in whatever way you can. But what if your doctors say, "There's nothing wrong with you," and the folks in your circle of family and friends believe the doctors and not you?

Okay, you want to put on a brave face and live your life. You can't deny that you're hurting, but others around you do, so you try to deny the pain. Maybe on some days, you want to believe that "what hurts" doesn't hurt so you can focus on what's happening around you rather than on how the pain is taking over. On those days, it's possible that you do even less—you can't concentrate at the office, so you muddle through about half your workload, or you just can't get out of bed. Then it comes: When you tell others how you feel, a stunning response knocks the breath out of you: No one quite believes you!

You know one thing: You're not asking for sympathy but for validation of a condition you know exists. Or you're calling on the expertise of the medical profession for answers, not for justification of the belief you have about your problem. Having this pain isn't strategic, a way to get attention or manipulate others' feelings about you. You haven't decided to feel pain; rather, it is truly physiological.

Self-doubt starts weighing into the equation, and you begin to think, "Am I crazy?" Why won't anyone believe that you really and truly feel the pain? You ask yourself the same question every day, seeking a way to live a fulfilling and pain-free life again.

When I see patients, I follow certain guidelines, beginning with the understanding that the patient's own report of pain is the best source of information. Then I immediately try to learn:

- How does the person talk about his pain?

- Is the person hesitant to admit to feeling pain? Can I get him to use other words to describe what he is experiencing?

- What else relevant to the pain is happening in his life that I should know about?

Terri's story is a great example: She'd had a benign but fairly large and rapidly growing tumor removed from an area behind her nipple, leaving a 1-inch scar and a slight discolored indentation. That was 3 years ago. Since she was worried about getting breast cancer, Terri was hypervigilant about every ache, pain, or odd sensation in her breasts. Every breast specialist assured her that she was fine and that the surgery left no "artifacts," or unusual conditions related to the surgery or the scarring. "I know what I feel," Terri insisted, "and that is shooting pains of varying degrees in my nipple a few times a week. Doesn't pain mean something, not nothing? I just don't get it. It makes me worry that I have a problem that isn't detectable or diagnosable. I sure don't like thinking that I'm making this up!"

Terri tended to be an emotional woman, but appropriately so. She wasn't a hysteric, and she had excellent coping skills. She was levelheaded and even helped take care of her elderly mother, who had a heart condition. Would Terri imagine pain? Not likely. Terri also experienced very severe migraines and injected herself every day with sumatriptan (Imitrex) without complaint or comment. Unless the migraine medication happened to not kick in, she didn't talk much about her headaches except to friends. At those times, she forced herself to function as best she could with intense headaches and not give in.

When I look at many of these people—whether they're like Terri, who is highly functioning, or like others, who are less so—I see people who are suffering. And not being believed adds to the ordeal. When I started in pain management, I found that the medicines or therapies prescribed by doctors were often the same, but the patients weren't. One size does not fit all. Everyone needs to be understood, and doctors need to take more time to do the understanding. You are a whole person, with a body, heart, and soul.

Talking about Pain with Your Doctor

When you feel physical and emotional pain, your doctor may be the first person with whom you let down your emotional guard. Since I see people who are in desperate need of help, it's not unusual for my first interview with them to begin with tears. When someone has been seeking a cure and has faced disbelief or disappointment from 6 or 10 doctors, I expect tears.

Tears make many doctors feel uneasy for any number of reasons. It's not that doctors are giving up on a patient or that they lack interest in treating her, but often they are uncomfortable due to their own unspoken sense of uncertainty or helplessness.

Arthur Frank, PhD, in an article called "How Stories Remake What Pain Unmakes," writes incisively and movingly about people dealing with pain. He raises the point that when people talk to their doctors, that communication is part of their relationship with each other. Ideally, doctors would encourage their patients to reveal feelings, or, in turn, patients would trust their doctors enough to talk without encouragement. However, most doctors and patients have a friendly but distant relationship in which the patient says one thing but means another—and hopefully, the doctor can see beneath the surface.

Dr. Frank writes that any patient in pain would like to "grab his or her physician in an arm lock and demand to know how to protect his or her life from the chaos of pain." The patient wants to corner the doctor and ask, "Will I get better?"—and get an absolute answer. But, Dr. Frank explains, doctors fear this kind of demand because they often can't answer such a question. Of course, a patient senses the doctor's fear and may end up fearing for herself even more.

Thus, the patient's story can have what seems to be an unhappy ending, punctuated by fear. This is the moment when I come in and encourage the patient's story to continue to unfold so that together we can seek a far more workable resolution.

Why We Can Disbelieve What's True

There are two other factors that contribute to disbelief: the way we learn to respond to infirmity and the way we learn to respond to others talking about their feelings. How we think about illness and how we think about revealing our feelings determine many of the effects that illness can have on us, and the same may be said about pain. As a culture, we're generally taught to ignore pain, to soldier on and push through. By stressing bravery and personal sacrifice, we regard those who are overcome by pain as weak and perhaps using pain as a way to be manipulative for their own interests.

If this is the thinking about others, what can we believe about ourselves? That having pain means we're self-indulgent and playing a game with others? I think not. I'll concede that there is a small percentage of pretenders who use illness as a weapon, but most people are sincere in their complaints.

Social influences also count. Many of us fear illness and don't like being around others who are ill. Fear of becoming sick and in pain can shorten our patience with others asking us for sympathy and answers. Those who are close to you may use denial as a defense— more a way of telling you they wish you were in perfect health than of implying you must feel no pain.

Men are still basically taught to control and suppress any feelings related to vulnerability, including pain and love, and to express emotions related to control, aggression, and anger. Even now, after the women's movement in the 1970s, women are generally raised to control aggression and anger and endure pain (especially childbirth) while also being taught that it is acceptable to express sympathy, fear, and love. So even though you may automatically feel one emotion or another, it has been conditioned, meaning it can be modified or un-learned! Feelings have no gender roles, and gender-role–related emotions you carry with you are not set in stone. Spiders inherit a blueprint for spinning a web and can't learn any pattern other than the one imprinted in their genes. Humans have the advantage of being conscious, able to examine their behaviors and beliefs and learn (and relearn) how to sweep away the cobwebs.

"Seeing" Pain versus Feeling It

When pain is real, though, why wouldn't a doctor believe you? It is probably the psychological "X" factor: Doctors can't quantify agony. There's no way to pinpoint pain on an x-ray or magnetic scan or to detect it in the blood. There's no device that uses electrodes or in-flatable cuffs to measure pain, although there are apparatuses that will determine if your heart is beating faster or slower, your breath is coming short, or your blood pressure drops. In fact, until the year 2000, pain was considered such an unreliable barometer of illness that it was not listed among the five vital signs doctors record dur-ing a patient's initial examination. The cruelest irony is that the symptom that most affects a patient is one most doctors don't know how to handle. If there's one reason for that, I'd say it is a lack of training. Only 7 percent of medical schools in America offer courses in pain management.

Then again, even *with* a medical education, some doctors dismiss complaints about pain from women, especially from endometriosis patients. Women with endometriosis often have terrible cramps before and during their periods, a fact of biology, not opinion. Historically, doctors did not give much credence to the pain wrought by advancing endometriosis. Instead, many doctors thought such women were "hysterical." Just such a woman once came to see me and started out by saying, "Please don't tell me I'm making this up!" She had low-grade pain from endometriosis all month, but the pain became increasingly severe during her cycle.

Vera was a working woman who ran an employment agency and who was totally involved in her sons' lives, but when the pain hit, she could not function. She'd bear up as much as possible, but then the crying would start and she'd often end up in the emergency room. After examining her, the doctors would tell her, "There's nothing wrong" and suggest she was a hysterical, depressed woman. Eventually, her husband became her advocate, arguing her case to doctors and insisting that Vera wasn't depressed, hysterical, or imagining the pain.

Here's the rub: Vera would get her pain medication when her husband was with her and insisted on it, but doctors didn't believe the extent of her pain when she went to the doctor without her husband. Even in the 21st century, it still is not unusual for women in pain to be disbelieved. Before she came to see me, Vera would wind up in the emergency room at least once a month. Now, she sees me for a checkup every month to check her progress and no longer has to go to the emergency room for medication. She's doing well, and her functioning is back to normal.

Fibromyalgia (FM), a pain syndrome that's fairly common among women but uncommon among men, may also stump doctors. There's no answer yet as to why it occurs; one belief is that it's a virus, and another suggests that it's related to hormone cycles. On the same spectrum as chronic fatigue syndrome, fibromyalgia creates pain in many different parts of the body at once. Fibromyalgia is thought to be a form of muscular rheumatism in which the person feels pain, soreness, tenderness, or spasms in the muscles, tendons, and ligaments. Interestingly, few people with the disorder experience it in exactly the same way. It can be difficult to diagnose, since many of the symptoms that make up FM can also exist by themselves. Doctors have been able to pinpoint only one definitive physical finding that's common to all people with FM: a sore or painfully tender feeling in some or all of 18 spots on the body. A criterion for diagnosis is that a patient experiences pain in at least 11 of those spots when pressure is applied to them.

Some women with fibromyalgia can be in pain much of the day or suffer intermittently, while others become totally dysfunctional. I treated a nurse who had the condition so severely that she became bed bound. Then, because she was bed bound with such severe pain, she became depressed because she couldn't work. Ultimately, I got her on a morphine-type drug that helped get her back on her feet.

Sadly, many people with fibromyalgia who are not bed bound feel hopeless, surrounded by their other problems. Beyond the pain, about 94 percent of people with FM have sleep disorders and awaken from restless sleep feeling stiff, tired, and achy. Others may experience dizziness, skin sensitivity, impaired coordination, and memory problems. And then we're back to a key question: What came first and what created what—depression or fibromyalgia? My concern is relieving pain, and I've discovered that antianxiety drugs don't help pain. However, a combination of modalities, such as a muscle relaxant to help people sleep and acupuncture treatments to alleviate the pain, can change the quality of life for people with pain.

Beginning the Healing Process

As I mentioned in Chapter 1, there are 75 million people who are affected at some time by chronic pain, yet there are doctors who dismiss it as being either imaginary or exaggerated. Interesting paradox! But there's another biological fact we have to consider: Chronic, persistent pain can change the way your body responds to a pain signal, so instead of developing an eventual tolerance to pain, your nervous system becomes increasingly sensitive to it. But believe me: No matter how sensitive you are to pain now or what your condition is, you can begin to heal by following the guidelines in this book.

The healing process has to begin with your assessment of your overall health in a different way, not just in relation to pain. To manage or significantly reduce pain, you must take the time to discover how you deal with getting through life day by day, with grief, with loss, with spirituality, and with the way you relate to others.

Why Am I Depressed?

You can be psychologically hurting and have physical pain, or it can start the other way around. "Am I depressed because of the pain, or is the pain worse because I'm depressed?" patients have asked me again and again. It doesn't matter what came first or where it started—it's still all part of the total pain picture. Most people don't need opiates or antidepressants but can benefit from taking a look in the mirror and facing themselves honestly. Most people don't need muscle relaxants but can benefit from exercise, which helps tremendously, or from acupuncture and other modes of complementary medicine.

My experience with pain patients tells me that many of them go through a confusion of feelings about their condition. This confusion can add to the initial stress of dealing with the pain and can lead to depression and any level of diminished ability to take care of responsibilities on a daily basis.

However, the truth is that there is an increase in pain for people who are depressed. In fact, depression may influence physical conditions in ways you might not have believed possible.

EMOTIONAL RESPONSES TO PAIN

For each statement, circle "T" if it is true or "F" if it isn't, regarding your emotional responses to pain.

- I worry that the pain will recur, and this makes me upset.   **T   F**

- I fluctuate between being angry about being in pain when it is at its worst and suffering from crying jags.   **T   F**

- When I have severe pain, I suddenly feel a loss of control over my body.   **T   F**

- I find that when the pain gets bad, I get severely depressed, which just makes the pain worse.   **T   F**

- Friends tell me I should seek help to deal with the pain, but the idea of going to a shrink makes me feel even more helpless.
  T   F

- I get very tired and can't concentrate because of the pain, but I continue to do what I can.   T   F

- I have to cancel plans at the last moment because I am not feeling strong enough or interested enough in going out. T   F

- I think my family tolerates my condition when the pain gets bad, but I secretly fear they see me as a burden.   T   F

- I know it can be hard for my friends and family to talk about how I feel and for them to sympathize with me.   T   F

- I am trying to sort out my feelings about my pain so I can let my friends and family know how much they mean to me. T   F

- I live in the present and try not to let past problems get in the way of enjoying life. I know that reliving events of the past in my head will not change them for the better.   T   F

- I know I am lovable and do not feel I have to do things for others so they will accept me and love me.   T   F

- I know my spouse/parents/children/boss/friends is/are not directly responsible for my pain.   T   F

- I do not blame my spouse/parents/children/boss/friends for any bouts of pain I may suffer or make them feel bad about what none of us can control.   T   F

- If I go to a pain management clinic or start pain management techniques, I would want someone close to me to join me for a few sessions.   T   F

- It would make me feel better to know someone close to me understands what I am going through.   **T   F**

- By being a perfectionist, I tend to place enormous pressure on myself. I am trying to accept my own shortcomings and give up some of the self-defeating thoughts that make me feel inadequate when I'm not.   **T   F**

Check how you're doing by tabulating your True and False answers. If most of your answers indicate a more positive attitude about yourself and your condition, this is very hopeful news for you. If most of your answers reflect a sense of defeat, now is the time to effectively get into gear and help yourself get well!

14–17 positive answers mean you're doing okay and are many steps ahead in getting your pain under control. Strive to understand the circumstances and feelings connected to any questions you answered negatively and figure out how to turn them around. Every time you eliminate negative feeling, you eliminate a problem.

10–13 positive answers indicate that you're getting by most of the time—but you still have unresolved problems related to your pain and would greatly improve with therapy. Take a close look at each negative answer you gave and analyze the issues. Don't hesitate to get professional help to break through the issues that are causing you emotional pain.

0–9 positive answers means that you can still help yourself, even if you are having bad days. You do best for yourself by being honest about your life and having a willingness to give up the emotional burdens weighing you down and adding to your physical pain. Talking to someone you trust about your emotional state and freeing yourself from emotional pain will make astonishing positive changes for you.

No matter what your score, I strongly suggest that you:

- Confront the issues that clearly cause mood change or depression for you.

- Seek assistance—unhesitatingly—when you need it.

- Learn to detach from the past and look ahead with a measure of optimism.

- Give yourself permission to ask for what you want and not play the victim.

- Be willing to try new techniques for pain control.

- Become an active partner in your health care so that pain no longer limits your chances for living a full and happy life.

Why Am I Feeling Stressed?

Your pulse and heartbeat quicken, your blood pressure rises, adrenaline pours into your bloodstream, and your body temperature may even rise. You have bouts of sleeplessness, and your diaphragm muscles tense, causing shortness of breath. No, you're not in love; you're responding physiologically to emotion-arousing stimuli that can short-circuit your productivity; make you susceptible to stress-related disorders such as chronic headaches, eating disorders, depression, stiff neck, backaches, and ulcers; and influence the severity of your pain.

I treat many patients whose pain either worsened or recurred during extremely stressful times due to personal or work-related conflicts. Stress is most definitely an active component of chronic pain, and patients who understand that they have control over their bodies and destinies are more successful when managing their pain. On the other hand, focusing on a sense of helplessness increases stress on the body, worsening pain.

What Negative Stress Does to You

Stress affects both body and mind. Tom, the businessman with knee pain whose story opens this chapter, found the effects of long-term stress to be devastating. Most of us can bounce back from a bad day at the office or at home, but we may be unable to do so if certain stresses continue day after day after day. In this situation, you can feel helpless or hopeless, tense or explosive, or you may act impulsively and without thinking of the consequences (think of road rage). Or you can feel exactly the opposite: You may have exaggerated fears of everyday acts, such as leaving the house or riding in an elevator.

The score in the health arena shows that stress is winning. According to the American Academy of Behavioral Medicine, which does extensive work on stress disorders and stress management, 30 million Americans have some form of major heart or blood vessel disease, 1 million have heart attacks each year, 50 million have high blood pressure, 8 million have ulcers, 14 million are alcoholics, more than 5 billion doses of tranquilizers are prescribed every year, and $15 billion is lost by American industry because of stress-related absenteeism.

Not *all* stress is unhealthy, however. Some stress creates challenges to compete, to invent, to run a marathon, or to adapt to situations. This is productive stress. But when stress is unproductive, it can contribute to your pain. Excessive worry over things you can't change, for example, creates negative emotional stress, or distress.

Let's get to Tom again: He was in what stress experts call the distress cycle, where pain stressors (his knees acting up) and emotional stressors (his anger response to the recurring pain) resulted in stress overload. It's the domino effect: The "causes" create stress overload, which can result in immediate or long-term problems. In Tom's case, there were heightened physiological responses, such as muscle tension and headaches, adding to a real medical disorder involving his kneecaps. The result: more pain, less pleasure in life, less enjoyment of his intimate relationships, and a misguided focus on work as a way to disconnect from what was really happening to his body. So although Tom's problem was from an old trauma, eventually it became aggravated by stress, causing more intense pain.

De-Stressing Your Life

Any attempt to de-stress your life has to begin with being kind to yourself, getting in touch with your spiritual side, maintaining a sense of humor about yourself and others, and giving up feeling like a victim. It helps if you do not see every word or deed in so serious a light. Try not to over-respond to the many situations you cannot change. The past is gone. What can be changed is how you react to events in your life.

Not every aspect of life has the same measure of importance. Your days have thousands and thousands of individual interactions, events, and episodes, and it is impossible to take them all in. To do so would be emotionally exhausting! However, many of us react or overreact to these moments, whether or not they are within our control, as if these events were all equally significant. They are not. An insignificant slight in the morning from your spouse or from a co-worker on the job need not set off a day-long chain reaction of self-defeating thoughts that can only lead to psychological and immune system stress.

Do you hear yourself reinforcing negative thoughts such as "I can never beat this problem," or "Why bother starting over at a new job? I'll never succeed," or "Everyone's got it better than me"? Listen to what you say to yourself and stop these thoughts. Replace them with positive thoughts about what you can do for yourself to improve your life. Selectively eliminate factors that, under objective scrutiny, turn out to be nothing but little disturbances.

A good attitude helps you feel more relaxed about life and connected to your place in the scheme of things. When you're stress free, your body's immune system can work more efficiently and effectively in relieving your pain.

Can How I Think Really Make a Difference in How I Heal?

Ending depression and de-stressing your life is complicated, but the healing that accompanies these actions is worth the effort. That means *your* effort, along with a support team to help you through. There is no magic box packed with the secrets of successful healing that you can open and use. Because of your unique perspective, experiences, and the situation of your life at this moment, your healing will not look or feel like anyone else's.

Knowing that life is limited forces you to look at yourself and ask what you are doing with your one and only life. And if you're in pain, the question is: Can this illness of yours be turned into a gift of knowledge rather than an ongoing crisis? Of course! In fact, I've developed an approach that helps patients examine who they are—from the minutiae of their everyday life to the chemistry of their bodies to how they experience spiritual awe—so we can treat the pain wherever we find it.

A good illustration of this is the way I worked with one of my pain and palliative teams with Ben, a 48-year-old construction worker.

Ben injured his back at a building site, and his doctors diagnosed a herniated disk. The recommendation for him was bed rest and epidural steroids, which are drugs injected directly into the spine to relieve the inflammation. These drugs didn't have much effect, and his doctors suggested surgery as a next step. Despite x-ray findings that showed that the surgery was technically successful, Ben's back pain persisted. At this point, he was suffering from what doctors call failed back surgery syndrome.

After nearly 5 years of excruciating pain and repeated futile trips to specialists, Ben was understandably depressed. His physician sent him to a psychiatrist, who prescribed antianxiety medication and antidepressants. These pills didn't relieve his pain or his sad state of mind, so his doctors sent him back into surgery. This time, they installed a dorsal column stimulator, a device attached to the spine that transmits electrical impulses to quell pain. Yet this surgery proved to be another disappointment: The device didn't do much good.

"Something else is wrong here," Ben said.

That's when I met him.

Ben is a type of patient I've seen frequently: someone who presents himself to the world as joyless, hopeless, stripped of energy, and looking as if misery were his faithful servant—even though he doesn't have a fatal diagnosis. Pain has done that to patients like this!

Ben was despondent and could barely walk the day he came to my clinic with his wife. I only had to ask how he felt for both of them to start sobbing. When we shifted the focus from the chronology of his treatments to his family medical history, the multiple sources of his pain became obvious to me.

Here's what happened: Eight months after he was injured, Ben's 24-year-old son and daughter-in-law died in a car crash, leaving Ben and his wife to care for the couple's twin infants. Two years after that, while Ben was in the middle of his unsuccessful treatments, his father died of a stroke, then his mother of a heart attack. The increasing severity of his back pain made it impossible for him to work, and he was forced to leave his company and go on disability. "I loved my work," he said, through wrenching sobs. "It was my life." Ben's wife, who hadn't worked for the duration of their marriage, but who had once worked as a bookkeeper, took a course to update her accounting skills and got an entry-level job to support the family.

One doctor saw the back pain. Another saw the depression. Neither of them saw the man.

For me, the first step in treating Ben was to get him on appropriate doses of medication so that he could deal with the physical pain. Once that was under control, we attacked his suffering. Although everyone has different core issues, the first step is the same for everyone: We must all shed our burdens. Everyone has them, but how we think of them and deal with them makes the difference. It was clear that Ben had many burdens—and that they were partly responsible for slowing his healing. But for him to shed them, he first had to accept and understand that he was carrying them. He needed to ask for help.

I asked the hospice clergy to work with Ben, telling the pastor,

"I've just found your project for the year." The pastor visited Ben at home and counseled him. With prayer and talking things out, Ben could finally grieve for and eventually celebrate the family he lost and spiritually reconnect with the family he still had. Dealing with many losses was only the first step, though. He also had to work on letting go of the past.

The sessions with the pastor were difficult for Ben, but they were immensely helpful for reorienting his thinking and his life. The next time I saw him, his eyes were brighter, and he seemed more optimistic. It was a sign that the healing process was on track. Ben was thinking about going back to work. I arranged to get him into a state-supported vocational training program for computer skills, a subject he tackled with incredible focus. Just having a purpose, a subject to wrap his mind around and apply himself to, was a huge distraction from the pain.

Ben completed the course and got a part-time job with his old employer, this time as a computer tech. This brought him back into the company he loved and gave him earning power in the household, thereby restoring some of his support network and his stature—surprise benefits of his new skill.

Without work, social contact, and the activities of daily living to give life structure and meaning, pain can be overwhelming. Ben is only one example of that. But life goes on, with new losses and difficulties. In many cases, chronic pain brings on financial troubles as bills mount and your income evaporates. You may think, "If I could get rid of this pain, my life would snap back in place. Everything would be perfect." Of course, life wasn't perfect before. When chronic pain enters the picture, we tend to romanticize the past and idealize our relationship to life. To really treat the pain, as with Ben, you have to comprehend and accept your losses as well as redefine an identity that is strong and vibrant within the limitations of your condition.

Believe You Can Make a Difference

What Ben's case demonstrates is a fundamental principle of healing: If we can't change a situation, we are challenged to change ourselves, as Viktor E. Frankl wrote in *Man's Search for Meaning*. After surviving the Nazi death camps, Frankl came to believe that the spirit of man is so strong, he can make meaning out of even the most terrible experience. We have no control over the things that happen to us, he wrote. We can only control our attitude toward them. Despite his unforgettable description of what he lived through, *Man's Search for Meaning* is a very optimistic book. Frankl urged his readers, as I urge my patients daily, "to say yes to life in spite of everything."

Attitude writes the script of life, and the most positive attitude is to say, "What can I do to stop the pain?"

When I hear a patient ask this question, I feel assured that the chances of relieving the pain are greatly improved. When you say this, too, it will tell me you're actively participating in your health care. And as a doctor, I know how much a positive attitude and active participation in your own healing can do to help you succeed. Sometimes, you need to accept that you may never have your old life back as it was, but it's important to remind yourself that you *do* have your life! Active participation means you can continue building a life in which you are still vital and connected to the world.

Taking charge of your pain involves change. There is no getting away from it. Change requires a real willingness to invest in yourself and alter some daily routines and ways of thinking about it.

This book takes on pain with a different set of ideas and perceptions than others you've seen before. The questions I want you to ask yourself will help you clarify your personal history with pain, while every therapeutic step I recommend can be healing and life affirming. I've seen miraculous changes, so I know these ideas have real power. I hope you will suspend your old beliefs and ideas about treating pain and where pain has taken you in the past. Be open to the techniques and approaches that can help reduce or heal your pain, and see what happens. Once you put aside the old beliefs that do not work for you and shift your thinking to what can work, your suffering will be reduced.

Keeping the Faith

We all live by faith—or "spirituality"—whether we're conscious of it or not. Faith gives purpose to life and adds meaning to actions. In its purest form, faith is so deeply felt that it explains why we do what we do. Faith touches the heart and the head. Most of us suffer or endure as long as we need to or want to, but once we change the intent of our thought—toward positive action—the suffering subsides. Change your thoughts, and you change your experience.

Some people, though, do not change their thoughts; they focus on the negative. In fact, many of them are preoccupied with feeling bad. This seriously impacts how they function and how they interact with others, and they are telling themselves that what they want for themselves is physical disorder and attention. Simply, their thoughts are not on having faith in the optimal functioning of their bodies, or in health, but on illness—physical or mental. And so they are rewarded: As they think they are, so they are.

Finally, let me leave you here with this story.

In my lectures on managing chronic pain, I like to tell the story of an elementary school teacher who asked her students to name the Seven Wonders of the World. Though there were some disagreements, Egypt's great pyramids, the Taj Mahal, the Grand Canyon, the Panama Canal, the Empire State Building, St. Peter's Basilica, and the Great Wall of China got the most votes.

After collecting the votes, the teacher noticed that one student hadn't yet turned in her ballot. She asked the girl if she was having trouble with her list.

"Yes, a little," the thoughtful girl replied. "I couldn't quite make up my mind because there are so many."

The teacher asked her to read her list aloud so the class could help her figure it out.

"I think the Seven Wonders of the World are to touch, to taste, to see, to hear, and to smell," she said, then hesitated before rounding out the seven. "And to laugh and to love."

Astonishing and profound. This is what I mean when I tell patients that chronic pain is healed through the senses. Conventional pain treatments try to dull the mind and the nerve endings. The patient doesn't feel the pain. In fact, she may not feel much of anything. As you go through this book, remember that pain is a sign that something *must* change. Severe pain is a call to action: to awaken your senses, to activate your values, to honor those you care about, and to express what you feel.

Do not shut down! If you continue to touch, taste, see, hear, smell, laugh, and love, you continue to live your own Seven Wonders.

CHAPTER 3

You're Not Alone!

How Pain Affects Your Relationships

. . . .

"I used to take my frustration out on my wife, even when she helped me out at work—as in, 'Why is she okay and I'm not?' I finally understand how much she does for me. I stopped hurting her because *I* was hurting!"

—*Jack, 28 years old*

"My life used to be about doing things and going places. We loved playing tennis, hiking, dancing. I'm not much past 40, but I feel like I'm old and holding my husband back because of my knee pain."

—*Nancy, 42 years old*

"Every time I ask anyone to help me, I feel guilty. I'm worried that *I'm* getting to be a real pain!"

—*Beth, 55 years old*

. . . .

These three very different people have very different stories to tell about how pain makes them feel, but each one is saying the same thing about how it impacts their lives at the deepest level—personal relationships. Jack dealt with pain through anger and aggression toward others until he saw how he'd unlovingly taken advantage of his wife. Nancy felt helpless about her pain, and she feared for her relationship with her husband. Beth worried about imposing on others, which she did not actually do.

If you have chronic pain, you know exactly what these three are talking about. Pain changes the nature of your relationships, sometimes making them closer and more intimate, sometimes causing distance, breakups, or loss. My hope for you is greater intimacy, but it takes a little thinking out to make mutual understanding more of a possibility.

Relationships are complicated to begin with, even when one of you is not in pain. Whether it's a love relationship with a spouse, partner, or child; a close friendship; a casual acquaintanceship; or association with your colleagues or health-care professionals, every relationship has a certain depth of attachment, feelings, a history, good and bad patterns of relating to each other, expectations, and responsibility to each other. The burden of pain disrupts intimate relationships, recreational activity, and employment—and it also profoundly shifts your personal and social role and therefore how you relate to others.

What can happen? For one thing, you may be the type of person who constitutionally prefers to withdraw from others when you're not feeling good—even until you've detached from a relationship. Your back hurts or your knees are so bad that you can't get in and out of seats easily, or your jaw pain is so bad that you can't eat, therefore, you won't go out to dinner and the movies with someone you care about. So you beg off and pretty much let others know you aren't available at all. And you tell them to go on without you. Are you being too hard on yourself? Are you isolating yourself when you needn't do so? Most probably! I've worked with patients who've retreated from others in one manner or another, and ironically, they don't feel better when they've shut themselves off from others. Instead, they feel even more alone.

Voluntary isolation and alienation are not good for the healing process! Neither is the reverse attitude, feeling and acting too much like a victim. While some people are stoics and say nothing, others do the opposite: They complain about their pain until others don't want to hear about it—friends, family members, spouses, and co-workers. I understand how either attitude can happen: Pain changes your opinion of yourself as well as your position in the family and in your social circle.

Good relationships, though, can help you take the focus off any sense of helplessness you feel so that you can heal. Negative relationships increase stress on your body, and as I discussed in the previous chapter, pain can worsen when stress is increased. The solution is to strengthen good relationships and, if necessary, distance yourself from destructive ones. For now, let's concentrate on the making of relationships and figure out how to make them better.

When You Feel Pain Is Your Partner

Joan, a patient, once said to me, "A few days ago, I believed that I'd be walking hand in hand into the future with endometriosis. Just the two of us, and good-bye to my boyfriend, getting married, having kids, and any sort of normal life." Clearly, this woman was suffering, and she hadn't yet tapped the source of her internal strength to cope, to go on, and to be sure she didn't sacrifice a good relationship to chronic endometriosis, a treatable disease.

In treating her, I discovered that Joan tended to talk about this menstrual disorder, and how medications did or didn't help, in moderation. She neither denied her illness nor tried to turn discussions to her problem no matter what the subject. Rather, Joan seemed reasonable. "If I had really bad cramps, I was more likely than not to break a date or make up an excuse to get home immediately after work," she said. She was also afraid that if she talked too much about endometriosis, her boyfriend would leave her, thinking she wasn't healthy and shouldn't be the mother of his kids. But there was the truth of the matter, too. "I was afraid that if I didn't tell him how bad my endometriosis was, he'd think I was okay and avoiding him—and that I didn't love him," she added. "Either way, I worried about what was going to happen."

Val, a former patient, also had endometriosis. I met her when she'd just broken up with her fiancé. Not wanting to believe it but saying it just the same, Val told me in what she thought was an aside, "I know my endometriosis drove Joe away. To me, what's terrible is having the man you're about to marry give up on you and walk out when you're sick and need him most. Joe was pretty much fed up with me and my condition and all our trips to the emergency room, occasionally in the middle of the night. I would double up with pain and feel like the wind was knocked out of me."

By not being correctly diagnosed as having endometriosis, some women endure unnecessary pain during their menstrual periods. It is not unusual to learn that such pelvic pain can become an overwhelming entity in itself, which can seriously stress relationships.

Val was such a case, having been misdiagnosed to begin with—doctors thought she had everything from venereal disease to a spastic colon to a bladder infection. Her severest bouts of pain lasted 3 or 4 days. After that, she'd feel achy, and then okay for most of the month. She casually told two office friends about her problem and made a weak joke about her cramps, which is when she discovered one of them was a fellow sufferer and that the condition had a name: endometriosis. Meanwhile, Val insisted, "Endometriosis destroyed my chances of marrying Joe. At least I learned what the pain was from and found a doctor who knew how to treat it."

Endometriosis can dramatically alter the daily rhythms of a woman's life. Coping with the disease not only requires fortitude of spirit, it also needs the understanding of others. Endometriosis is not PMS, but it is one of those diseases that can mystify doctors.

What's thought to happen is that menstrual blood that doesn't flow out of the body in a normal manner can back up into the abdominal cavity. The backing up eventually wreaks far greater havoc than just causing menstrual cramps. It can lead to endometriosis when renegade endometrial cells attach themselves to an organ—

bowel, fallopian tubes, ovaries, or bladder—and grow with each monthly cycle. However, neither hormonal fluctuations during menstruation nor cramps necessarily signal the existence of endometriosis. What's more, many women who are spared monthly cramps go through life blissfully unaware that they have the disorder. For these women, endometriosis is diagnosed when they complain of painful symptoms other than menstrual cramps, when they discover that they cannot conceive, or when they miscarry.

Because endometriosis is so variable in nature, it can cause all sorts of complications, severe pain being only one symptom. Physical pain doesn't exist in a vacuum; generally it results in a life-changing state of emotional distress—a devastating side effect made worse by the belief among others—doctors, family, or friends—that the pain doesn't exist or couldn't be "that bad."

Does Pain Itself Keep People Away?

It's always sad when couples break up or friends move on when pain is a very present third party. But is it pain that drives people off? Yes and no. I've seen many patients with cancer surrounded by people at a stage when they have the most pain. In this case, the existence of pain doesn't keep people away; in fact, it is an element that draws them closer. People are more tolerant of another's pain when they know the person is close to death. Also, there's an expectation that it is okay for people with cancer to complain, but that it's less okay for someone with a non-life-threatening condition to do so. How people respond to you when you're in pain will always depend on your own attitude toward it. So, yes, people are more tolerant when pain is life threatening, but when it's not, they may question your degree of misery. If you're the one in pain, the question, "Are you really hurting that bad?" is not what you want to hear.

Staying Connected to Others

I want to help you avoid viewing yourself as a victim of chronic pain or of a devastating disease and instead take charge of strengthening old relationships and forming new ones with those you feel for or love—including those in your social or work circles. When you take this step, you learn to tune in to other people's expectations of what you can and cannot do. There are many ways of asking for what you need, just as there are many ways to discuss clearly, without anger or compromise, how you want to be treated.

Most of all, you need to stay connected to the world through others. Stay connected to the good relationships and, if necessary, distance yourself from or terminate the bad ones. If you help build and sustain good relationships—even during your time of pain—no one will leave you. Instead, they'll rally around.

So, who's important in your life? Whom can you trust? Who would not be there if you needed someone in an emergency?

Examining the Nature of Your Relationships: Questions to Ask Yourself

I'm going to ask you to read through the following questions, which relate to the people in your life, and write down your answers. If you skip over a question because you're unsure of the answer, go back and think about it. It's important to get a true perspective on how you feel and what your relationships are to others.

Let's start with your support system.

WHOM CAN I TRUST?

• Do you feel loved?

_____

_____

• Are you married/divorced/widowed/single?

_____

• Do you have children?

_____

• Do you have pets?

_____

• With whom do you live?

_____

• Do you believe you are getting emotional support from your family?

_____

_____

• Do you feel close to your friends?

_____

_____

• Are your friends supportive?

_____

_____

• Do you think you are communicating effectively with your friends and family about your illness?

_____

_____

• Who is your main support?

_____

_____

• Do you feel close to the person who is your main support?

_____

_____

• Do you think this person understands what you are going through?

_____

_____

• Are you satisfied with your sex life?

_____

_____

• Whom do you see regularly?

_____

_____

• On whom can you depend?

_____

_____

• Whom do you trust?

_____

_____

- Who validates your point of view?

_____

_____

- Who seems rushed and distracted when you describe your condition?

_____

_____

- With whom are you fighting?

_____

_____

- Are there some relationships you consider to be a burden?

_____

_____

- Is anyone retreating from you?

_____

_____

COPING AND PERSONAL STRESS— MANAGING YOUR PERSONAL LIFE

The following series of statements looks like a "true or false" quiz. But don't be fooled by appearances—this questionnaire is a little more involved than it appears. Answer whether you "agree" or "disagree" with each statement. If you agree, think of an example of that situation and write it down.

For example, agree or disagree with the statement, "People say that I never actually tell them what I want or think, but I hint around or make suggestions. I don't understand why I need to go into great detail all the time."

If you agree, what do you say to people when they ask you how you feel?

One patient of mine answered this way: "I can't look very good since I'm not sleeping too well, my back is killing me, and the doctor said I have to stop smoking. Don't ask if I'm climbing the walls! I don't really feel like making a list of what I need and hoping people will get it or do it for me. You just have to look at me to know I need some help!"

How revealing this was. This patient was overly judgmental about herself, and she wanted people to guess what she needed without her telling them. This was asking a lot of others, who were not mind readers and not able to be supersensitive to her pain. This woman felt very unsure of others and was probably afraid she'd be rejected when asking for help.

Try to give detailed answers. The more you understand about why you're feeling pain, and the more you understand how you respond to others, the better off you will be.

- People say that I never actually tell them what I want or think, but I hint around or make suggestions. I don't understand why I need to go into great detail all the time.

_____

_____

- I have a feeling that no matter what I do, life for me will remain the same.

_____

_____

• I worry about being a good person and whether others think well of me.

_____

_____

• I would say that most of my friends and relatives are tired of hearing me talk about my pain.

_____

If the answer is "yes," the reason is (circle one):

(a) I tend to bring the subject around to my pain no matter what we're talking about originally, and it bothers them.

(b) I'm unsure if others really believe how much I'm in pain, so I emphasize it.

(c) I'm upset that they're okay while I'm limited because of my pain, so it's my way of letting them know how lucky they are.

(d) It's tough for people who care about me to hear about my pain, not wanting to know how I feel is one way they protect themselves.

• I'm very dependent on my husband/partner/parents/children and worry about being on my own, especially with my pain problems.

_____

_____

• When I'm angry, depressed, or lonely, it's easier to turn to chocolate or sugary foods for comfort than to express my feelings.

_____

_____

- I've lost interest in sex and worry that because of my chronic pain, my libido is gone forever.

- I live in the present and try not to let past problems get in the way of enjoying life.

- I'm working on giving myself permission to relax, or relax more often.

- I no longer have unrealistic expectations about my husband/partner/parents/children and try to accept them as they are.

- If I ever need to go to a pain management clinic, I would want my significant other or a good friend to join me in at least one session. It would make me feel better to know they understand what I'm going through.

- When I need a supportive person to help me through a difficult bout of pain, I know whom to call. This person is totally on my side and is never undermining or negative.

Your Family History

We are all the products of our genetics, our upbringing, the life experiences that were foisted upon us, and the experiences we chose for ourselves. I have seen many patients who respond exactly as their parents would to pain or even to a need for medical attention. Many times, mother, father, and child are all panicky, hysterical, sober, stoic, or moderate. Even when you're grown up and able to make your own choices, you may respond to illness in a way that may hold you back from healing.

What I'd like you to look for in your answers about your family are *any* attitudes that indicate a defeated, self-deprecating point of view about yourself that you've carried with you from the past. Can you pinpoint where a diminished ability to cope with the stresses related to pain might have originated? One of the benefits of examining your family relationships is that you can examine your family's health legacy. When you find a negative attitude that does not serve your best interest for healing, do what you can to stop acting on it.

Take Amy's case. Amy was a patient with fibromyalgia who told me after answering these questions, "These are issues I never thought about, since all I could think about was the pain and how to stop it. I had to face some of the feelings I tried to bury. I grew up with a mother who was terrified of doctors and made a huge fuss whenever she had to take me or my brothers to see one. When I told her about being diagnosed with fibromyalgia, she went into a panic. I see how her hysteria has always been contagious! I can see why I believed other people don't want to know about my condition. I'm afraid of upsetting them, and of them upsetting me. Now I want to make others part of my healing and stop disconnecting who I am from others."

Because the definition of "family" is different for everyone, answer these questions as they apply to you. Generally, by family, doctors usually mean "nuclear" family, which includes parents and siblings and, if you're married, your spouse and children. If your version of family is "extended" family, which includes aunts, uncles, cousins, and grandparents, then include them in your answers as well.

- Is there a history of depression in your family, treated or untreated?

_____

_____

- If some of your family members have died, what was the cause?

_____

_____

- What kinds of relationships did you have with them?

_____

_____

- Are you estranged from any members of your family?

_____

_____

• Are there episodes with your family that you regret?

_____

_____

• What was your family's coping style when you were growing up? (Circle one.)

    (a) Were your parents generally positive or negative about the ups and downs of life? Could they deal with unexpected events by seeking solutions and adapting to change without panicking?

    (b) Did either parent basically see the glass as half empty rather than half full?

    (c) Did your parents reach out to others and have friends, or were they suspicious of others, preferring to isolate themselves?

• When there was a health problem, did either parent react with extreme alarm or feel victimized? Or were they reasonable and capable, and did they act appropriately?

_____

_____

• Were your parents able to express affection to you and show their feelings in general? Or were they reticent and prone to keeping their feelings hidden?

_____

_____

Making Connections

Often, pain and other people don't mix.

I'm not going to kid you here. There will be times when the pain will be overwhelming and days when it will be hard to get out of bed. You won't want anyone around you, or you'll want everyone to automatically know what you need and get it for you without your having to ask. But people may be as important as any treatment, medication, therapy, or drug. When you're in pain, nothing replaces a good relationship with others you can trust, who can accept you and offer comfort. But just as important is your ability to understand and accept what those people can and cannot give you. Taking others into your confidence and accepting them as they are can bring you greater self-understanding, psychological relief, and closer relationships than ever.

To me, relationships always come first. As I mentioned earlier, I have a high pain threshold and can function pretty well with migraines or back pain from a herniated disk. However, I've trained myself to put pain to the side, so to speak, and move through the day at work, come home, and take care of my family as best I can. Or I may excuse myself from the dinner table if I'm really exhausted and achy in order to turn in early. I try not to make my pain the main focus, so that my co-workers, friends, husband, and children don't feel uncomfortable or denied their needs. It's not always easy when the pain is bad, and I'm not always perfect, but I keep trying because I trust that my family will always come through for me.

Others, I know, have different sensitivity levels and distinct coping styles and are flattened by headaches, endometriosis, carpal tunnel syndrome, arthritis, fibromyalgia, or other such pain-inducing disorders. Remember: The intensity of pain you feel varies by cause and location. But inevitably, your interpretation of the pain, or how you cope with it, makes the difference in your healing process. Other people are part of that coping equation.

That important, trusting give-and-take in relationships is possible for everyone. We've got to stop rushing around for a minute and think about our connections to others we care about and who care about us. As a culture, we've lost some of the capacity to take care of ourselves. Our world is set up so people are always on the run, busy with goals, worrying about money, jobs, the kids, the future. And there is always some kind of toll on us, such as a temporary or permanent loss of health or the toughest loss to bear, losing someone we love or have become attached to.

Medical professionals face deep loss on a daily basis. I spend a good part of the day with people who are great distances from their families and in severe pain. In a very real way, doctors and nurses fill the roles of friends and family for these people. We let them know they're not alone, and they come to trust in us.

When doctors see a patient in extreme pain, we feel it, even if we don't let the patient see it. We need to be comforting and minister to them as professionals. And if we lose a beloved patient, we feel it but rarely discuss how we feel! The toll this takes on us is heavy—a relationship that was important is gone. In addition, there are the everyday pressures of working at a hospital, doing what we can to ease the pain of the living.

I decided to find a simple way to defuse some of the tensions that all my colleagues went through every day at a hospital. My solution: I established a tradition with my staff of having lunch with them every day promptly at noon, no excuses. We sit at a table in my office with real silverware, napkins, good dishes, and home-cooked food provided on a rotating basis by the members of the team. I guess it's a staff version of my tea party for patients. At first, there was some grumbling about conforming to a schedule, but that rapidly changed: The feeling that lunch was an obligation was transformed into the creation of a closer team. Real connections. Trust. Lunch became a situation where we could understand and express our own feelings of loss or grief and have the other team members acknowledge the sacrifice and commitment of caregiving. Lunch is our own place to heal.

As a result, I've always got food in the office: leftover chicken curry or some delicious soup, along with muffins, brownies, or homemade cookies stashed around my desk. After I'd been at the job a few months, word got around that food could be found in my office. Doctors seemed to hover around my desk every afternoon. First they'd start by asking if I had something to nibble on or if there were any brownies left. My policy is to always stop whatever I'm doing if an actual person with a real problem is standing in front of me. Phone calls, e-mails, or a budget review can always wait. I'd rummage around and find some goodie, and then the real purpose of the visit would come out: One young doctor worried that she'd chosen the wrong specialty, while another confessed how bad he felt for one of his failing patients, a sentiment that usually is not shared with other professionals. I realized I wasn't just palliating the patients; the staff needed healing, too.

I tell you this about my practice in the hope that you will understand that your doctor counts as an important person in your life, and not just as the provider of medical care. Most of all, I hope to show you that doctors care, but we need to be self-protective, too. We see patients when they are in need of help, and very rarely when they are healthy. To keep functioning at our best and provide the best care for you, we have to disconnect just enough from our emotions.

I also tell you this because the act of extending yourself just a little to others, with or without a stash of cookies, works wonders. When you can create an environment of trust, where you can say what you feel and know that others respect you for it, it is one of the greatest relationship-bonding steps you can take.

Helping Yourself Heal

Remember, any change in your life has to begin by being kind to yourself, maintaining a sense of humor about yourself and others, and giving up the feeling of being life's victim. Try not to take every word and deed in too serious a light and try not to over-respond to what others say and do. When you judge yourself by whether or not you get another's approval, you make their opinion of you more important than what you think of yourself.

On the other hand, self-approval builds a good attitude, and a good attitude indicates a stronger sense of self-esteem. Self-esteem allows you to express realistic doubts and fears to others about how you feel, without a morbid overlay of doom. Many people go through a confusion of feelings about being in pain and what the condition means in terms of living a long and healthy life. This confusion can add to the stress of dealing with pain, a diminished ability to take care of responsibilities on a daily basis—and the additional stress of needing another's help. The circle closes.

Needing others is part of the human condition. We get into trouble when the person we need can harm us more than help us.

Identify Damaging Relationships

Sometimes, whatever pain you have can be exacerbated by a bad relationship. I treated a woman who came to us with an underlying illness that could not be diagnosed at first. Sally's symptoms were severe headaches that, she said, prevented her from fully functioning. An anesthesiologist I worked with realized that Sally had occipital neuralgia, a simple kind of muscular disorder where the muscles in the back of the neck get really tense and inflamed. To treat her, he injected the area with local anesthetics, which helped clear up the pain. But Sally was back the following week, complaining of serious pain in her left ankle that, she said, had bothered her slightly for years. Suddenly, it was so agonizing that she couldn't walk without limping badly.

I thought that her ankle problem was some sort of reflex sympathetic dystrophy, in which the tendon cords in the back of her foot were tight, and that she might have aggravated the nerve. We did some tests, and I told Sally to come back in a few weeks. She surprised us and turned up sooner, without an appointment—and crying hysterically. This was a tip-off to us that Sally was suffering a lot, and from more than just physical pain.

After calming down, she told us that she'd just moved from Oklahoma to the Washington, D.C., area with her husband 6 months earlier. Sally was working in sales at a large department store and was relatively happy at her job. However, after 2 years of marriage, Sally discovered that her husband, Don, had dipped into their savings without telling her and made a bad investment. Except for $100, all the money was gone. The man she thought she'd spend her life with, the man she trusted, proved himself to be not only dishonest with her but also irresponsible.

Panicky about money, Sally confessed that she felt like a "total mess" because of her body pains, and she was stressed because of her strained relationship with Don. She said that Don was otherwise a caring man, and he always did what he could to make her feel comfortable at home when she was in pain.

Sally and Don needed to solve their marital issues. I recommended a therapist, which is part of our program. At first, Sally didn't connect the changes in her relationship with her pain, and she had no idea that they mattered. She wanted Don to remain the good guy, but meanwhile, she feared that he wasn't. She was hurting, literally. Finally, she got the connection, but she still blamed herself. Taking their money behind her back was "bad stuff," but she told me, "I feel guilty, like I should have listened closer about him wanting the money. He said he didn't want to worry me, with this going on a year or so. Maybe it's true. Maybe I was so wrapped up in my own problems, Don did what he had to."

Sally was still making excuses for her husband, which was not a healthy attitude for her to take. She was adding to her physical pain by beating up on herself, taking the blame when it was Don who should have owned up to his dishonesty and duplicity. Don may have needed the money, but what he needed more was to grow up and take responsibility for his actions. My hopes for Sally were that she would see Don for who he was, stop downplaying her pain, and allow herself to heal.

So whom can you trust? Which relationships can be counted on and which are doing you harm? How do you let go of those who are harming you and move on so you feel free, not dazed from the loss? Unfortunately, there's no absolute formula that tells you what constitutes a perfect relationship when pain is a third party. There are guidelines, though, that make sense and help you examine your key relationships.

Before we go to the next chapter, where I'll go deeper into the process of releasing the psychological burdens of people and situations that add stress and emotional pain to your life, there are a number of important steps you can use right now to improve your relationships. Each step is meant to help you break the cycle of feeling alone or misunderstood, help you clarify how you and the people in your life relate to each other, and, critical to the mix, encourage you to appreciate others and build your self-respect.

Step 1: Give Up Fantasies about Being Rescued

It's not uncommon to wish that someone wonderful, with resources and curative powers, will meet you, fall for you, move into your life, and take over your care or take you away from your pain. Sure, it may happen, but the chance of a rescue miracle is slim. These dreams actually leave you feeling more frustrated with what others really do for you, as well as increase your feelings of being let down and limited. Rescue yourself from such thoughts. You do more for yourself when you pull your own weight in your own care rather than put all your hopes on someone doing it for you. When you let go of the rescue fantasy, you leave yourself free to seek every possibility for pain relief.

Step 2: Deal with Any Depression

This is one of the biggest problems with pain patients, and it's a significant cause of troubled relationships. A counselor can help you articulate your feelings, help you understand how depression affects you and the people around you, and show you what you can do to lift your spirits.

You must face depression and get help.

Think about what depression does to you. It breaks down your immune system, your brain becomes logy so your thinking is foggy, and you become hypersensitive. Depression can lead you into isolation, where something else happens that's not good for you emotionally: You expect less and less of yourself.

I spoke with Sonya Friedman, PhD, the bestselling author of a number of self-help books and a psychologist in Birmingham, Michigan, about the problem. She told me right off, "The first thing to do is always deal with depression. Don't give in to it or get to the point where you want other people to do things for you because you cannot function. That kind of surrender further inhibits healing. Instead, you have to resist surrender, and fight."

How do you resist? Rather than checking in with how you feel, check out what's in your best interest. There's a crucial distinction between the two. For example, suppose a friend says to you, "I'll pick you up in an hour and take you out to lunch. You don't have to do anything—I'll drive and you choose the spot." If you're depressed and answer, "I don't really *feel* like getting dressed, and it's too hot out, and I don't want to be around people in a restaurant," such a response is *not* in your best interest.

Move those negative feelings aside. "It doesn't matter how you feel," Dr. Friedman says. "Would you only do your job, or lose weight, or exercise, or even get therapy just when you *feel* like it? No." What matters is that you figure out what's in your best interest and program in all the things that are good for you.

Depression is manageable. Finding out what you can do for yourself will help both you and those around you.

Step 3: Be Honest with Others about Your Pain

One of my patients, with serious arthritis and a knee replacement, was one of the most stoic people I've ever met. That is, until the pain in his legs got brutal. Vic told me that he used to feel bad about feeling bad around his wife, until he finally accepted the fact that on some days, pain flattened him. "I may not be able to walk across a room or stand up for more than 2 minutes," he said, "but we still have a life. At those times, my wife does what she can for me. This includes buying movie tickets while I sit in the car, so I don't have to stand in line. I feel lucky that she understands what I'm going through and does what she can to make my life easier. Strangely enough, with all the problems with my bones, I feel lucky that what I have isn't life threatening, at least not yet! We remind each other of that every day."

Vic and his wife created a lifestyle that gave him permission to do less of certain things—to lie down when he needed to—and be honest with people about his condition and limitations. Vic's wife was not shy about reminding him that he shouldn't push himself beyond his physical limits on some days by, say, playing a few extra holes of golf. She said that not paying attention to what would help him meant that he was contributing to his own discomfort. Mostly, Vic said, "we talk about the alternative—living a very high quality life even though I'm in some sort of pain every day."

Since relationships extend beyond your home, be as honest as you can with your co-workers and employer, too. Vic said that he used to be proud of how well he hid his pain from his co-workers and boss, but it was at a huge toll to his health. As a company manager, Vic had to do a lot of standing and walking around, which knocked him out at the end of the day. Finally, when he could barely make it to his car because of his pain, he told his boss. Because the boss liked him, he shifted some procedures around so Vic could cut down on time spent on his feet.

If you have chronic pain, let your boss or partners know exactly what your problem is. What's best is for you to stay on the job. Once you've quit work, you lose the routines, the social interactions, the paycheck, and whatever degree of satisfaction you get from accomplishments on the job. You leave the normalcy of life. We've found that patients who do leave tend to struggle more because they feel isolated at home during the day.

This brings up another question: Are employers sympathetic, or are they more likely to find your health problem bothersome? Most employers can't afford to be sympathetic to those who are out too often. If you can function with back pain, migraines, or fibromyalgia, and you hit a point where you feel you can't go on, let me suggest this: See if you can make an arrangement with your boss that you can stop and rest for 15 minutes until you're closer to okay and able to continue to do your job. This builds your confidence and keeps you going. The point is to keep you working if you do not have to take too many days off.

Most of all, it's about being honest so that you can work with and around the pain—and around others.

Step 4: Be Honest about What You Want from Others

I've listened to patients talk about this issue, and almost everyone asks me, "How do I tell my husband/wife/partner/friend/child what I need at that moment? What if I'm imposing on them? What if I want them to leave me be and maybe check in later?" Some people have a difficult time with communication; they feel uncertain or embarrassed about saying what they want, but telling others what you need from them is really easier than you think.

Always tell the people who are there to help you that you're happy to see them. A comment like, "Thanks for coming," or "Thanks for checking on me. I'm glad you're here," acknowledges them in a very comforting and confidence-building way. You've made personal contact with them, and they'll be willing to help you without feeling as if you are taking advantage of them.

Then again, if a friend or relative helping you is not doing what you need or want, let that person know in a kind and direct statement. You could say something like, "Thanks, but I don't want any dinner now. I'll eat later. But I'd love to take a nap for an hour or so." Remember, people who are there to help have good intentions. Being demanding or angry at them for not being able to mind-read hurts the relationship and makes both of you feel bad. Similarly, if someone offers to help you in a way that's totally wrong for you, curb the impulse to be sarcastic. A remark like, "If you don't know by now, I won't tell you," is your pain talking.

Another variation of this behavior is to be uncommunicative and not respond to simple questions like, "Do you want another pillow? A cup of tea?" Not really listening, not responding, or showing no interest in what a helpmate is saying to you is destructive behavior. Being silent or tossing them a displeased look doesn't help you or the relationship.

Ultimately, when you communicate honestly with others and acknowledge them, you also acknowledge your own needs. It can only benefit you.

Step 5: Resist Isolation — You Need Others around You

I spoke about the undermining effects of isolation earlier, and I want to emphasize it here. Resist it! For some people, chronic pain means eventual detachment. Initially, friends and family will try to encourage you to socialize, but they may back down when they feel that you're trying to separate from them. I understand that immobilizing pain can mean you stop going to work or out on social engagements, but soon, people will stop asking you.

Truly, isolation can be deadly, so get yourself a weekly planner and start writing in social activities. Seek out a support group of other people who are in chronic pain. This can help you recognize that you're not different, and neither are they. Most important, you'll be around others. Allow yourself to laugh, and even laugh at yourself. You can also find mentors at these groups who offer some promising ideas for feeling better.

One of my patients, a 45-year-old woman going though an emotionally difficult time because of a recent divorce, also had arthritis. After much coaxing, Fran began attending a support group for people with arthritis. She was able to ask herself, "Am I better if I have things to do instead of concentrating on the pain?" The answer was yes. At a group session, she learned of a cherry concentrate that someone said could help ease the arthritis pain. Fran told me, "For all I know, it's a placebo. But I can tell you I've been feeling better since I started it over the course of 3 weeks."

What's important is that Fran got herself out. She learned to be open to people making suggestions to help her feel better, and she tried them. Very often, when you're in pain, you don't want to try anything. It's important not to identify yourself with your disease, so you can really live your life.

Getting involved in someone else's life in a sincerely interested way, or in activities at home such as gardening (try indoor gardening on a tabletop if the weather or your condition prevents you from bending or kneeling outside), takes the focus off the pain. The important thing is to find and maintain connections with some activity you like or someone you like. These connections can be found anywhere—in nature, in art, or with other people.

Step 6: Keep a Journal

Because pain can play havoc with your emotions, I suggest you keep a journal to help you vent your feelings. You can feel released from stress when you write down how you feel, how others respond and react to you, what you say to them, what they have or have not done for you, what you look forward to, what you think you've missed, or what you believe is lost to you. A journal is for your eyes only. It's one of the most creative ways to express your feelings on paper rather than taking them out on someone around you.

Your journal can be anything made of paper—a spiral-bound notebook, a hard-bound, cloth-covered book with blank pages, or sheets of paper stapled together. Don't worry about your writing style or your handwriting. Treat yourself to a pen that expresses your personality or your mood. I had a patient who wrote about her problems with fibromyalgia in red ink, about her husband in blue, and about her son in green.

Only you can create the true portrait of your life, with color, texture, feeling, spontaneity, and joy. Others are part of that. Draw them in and keep them closer to you. Since life is short; feel gratitude that you have made it to this point with others who care about you and whom you care about. Most of all, trust in your courage to make life better now for yourself. Call or visit a friend or family member today. Love is a painkiller!

what you can do to help yourself now

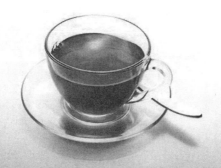

CHAPTER 4

Tapping Into the Miracle of Spirituality

How Deep Inner Connections Help End Your Sense of Feeling Like a Victim

What do live chickens, humor, inner peace, and a connection to the power of spirituality have to do with healing your pain? Everything!

This is why: In the weeks before I changed jobs from one big medical center to another, my appointment book was jammed. In addition to my regular caseload, former patients were calling to see me one last time. Some wanted final advice for their continuing pain management, while others just wanted to thank me for my care and to bid me good luck in Bethesda.

During an especially difficult day in this hectic transition period, I was in the hospital oncology ward when my pager went off. I called the number and heard the frantic voice of the office receptionist saying, "Dr. Berger, we have a problem—a *situation* in the waiting room."

My mind immediately raced through images of patients in distress. I was about to ask, "Which patient and what situation?" when the receptionist continued with, "One of your patients has brought in a chicken!"

"Is it cooked?" I asked.

"No, it's alive. And it's racing around the waiting room," she answered, sounding more than frazzled.

"I'll be right there," I promised.

I got there minutes later and saw Debbie, a young woman patient of mine—a farmer by profession—who had first come to the center's clinic a year before with full-body pain her doctors could not treat effectively. After a few appointments and tests, I determined that the source of Debbie's pain was undiagnosed multiple sclerosis. I referred her to a specialist and devised numerous therapies, both physical and spiritual, to help her manage the pain. That day, Debbie was fulfilling her longstanding pledge to introduce me to Lola, her pet chicken—the animal who, she told me, had been a great source of comfort to her during the difficult early stages of her pain management.

"Debbie!" I said gleefully, as I gathered up the blanket that she'd wrapped around the squirming brown-and-white bird. Lola, squawking wildly in these unfamiliar and antiseptic surroundings, was losing feathers that were flying everywhere, and the whole waiting area was in an uproar. Then my soon-to-be ex-boss walked by and stopped, and his jaw dropped. He smiled, shook his head, and said, "Annie, maybe the world is not ready for you!"

What this pet chicken meant to Debbie in healing power also meant something to me as a doctor of pain management: Here was a woman who tapped into interconnectedness to another creature and found solace and pleasure at being in the presence of the bird—and she allowed that connection to help alleviate her pain so that she could carry on her life as fully as possible. I believe that people create the emotional meaning of their pain and that they cope with the stress and reality of physical and emotional pain in their own ways. If a patient's source of comfort is a pet chicken, why should I suggest that her choice makes no sense because I would not make that choice for myself?

My techniques and approaches to healing pain may sometimes be unconventional, but traditional medicine backs me up regarding the positive effects of spirituality for patients suffering with pain and illness: It works, it's necessary, and it makes a difference—no matter if that spirit is found within religion, an image of God, a higher power, nature, art, sports, crusading for others' rights, wildlife, or barnyard creatures.

Remember: How you think reflects back on you and helps establish an accurate picture of how you live, and that also means how you live with pain. Let me contrast what Debbie has done for herself with Rob, a patient who said he never wanted to put himself out there in the work world and compete. Besides this fear, Rob admitted that he didn't like the actual exertion it took to achieve at a job, nor did he have any interest in finding his version of job satisfaction. He was disappointed in himself, yet his ambitions were nil, and his emotional dynamics were immature: He pretty much wanted to stay home and have his wife support him.

What happened? Rob began having chronic and serious knee problems, a result of an old high school football injury. He had to quit his salesman's job, where he stood up most of the day, and retire to his couch.

Because he was unemployed, his family was having a hard time financially. Rob walked with a cane, when he could walk. He had an agile intellect, which meant he could do some computer work from home for income, but his life was focused on his disability, his suffering, and his pain. This was the life Rob chose, and he came to believe that bad knees were God's punishment. By saying to himself over and over, "I don't want to work because I'm suffering," he essentially helped make chronic knee pain a constant in his life. Rob was spiritually turned off, focused on his suffering rather than on healing his body and his soul, and not growing up. The philosopher who said that men will give up almost anything but their suffering sadly had a man like Rob in mind.

Who of the two will do better in the long run? Obviously, it will be Debbie, who is above all spiritually intact, even though her illness is more serious than Rob's. Who is suffering more? Clearly, Rob.

Spirituality—It Could Be Your Key to Healing

Patients always ask me why I bother talking about spirituality with them. "Is it really important?" they ask. "Just give me the medication and I'll be fine," they insist. I tell them, "Spirituality is the *most* important aspect in healing." I'm not alone in thinking this. A scientific poll found that 79 percent of respondents believe that spiritual faith can help people recover from injury, illness, or disease. Your psychological makeup and social, intimate, and work dynamics are components of getting better, but spirituality touches on three key issues for all of us: meaning-of-life issues, life transitions, and, to use familiar terms, the state of one's soul. Thus, physical healing isn't fully possible without spiritual healing.

What Is *Spirituality?*

A patient checked in recently for a bone marrow transplant, knowing he'd have to be confined to a hospital bed for at least 100 days. Todd loved mountain climbing, rafting, and other outdoor sports that required skill and physical prowess. His life was now on the line. He said that being indoors for over 3 months would be the toughest thing he'd ever have to do, since he felt his "heart was anywhere there were rocks and flowing water"—but what choice did he have? Todd took good advice from a clinic chaplain, and he arrived at the hospital with a stack of picture books on rafting and mountaineering. This allowed his mind to be transported to the places that made him feel whole. He could also meditate on the images when he needed comfort.

Is this spirituality? Absolutely! Did Todd manage his pain and pull through? Happily, he did.

Spirituality is a personal experiential connection with the universe that is larger than you and is in, through, and around you. Spirituality is both deep and wide—and it is many things. Without it, we yearn for "something" to fill an inner core. With it, anything is possible. The power of spirituality is that it is affirmative, uplifting, and motivating. If you're in pain, this power eases the suffering. In my experience, people who have a more difficult time with pain don't have spiritual beliefs.

Spirituality involves finding that soul-filling center in making art, playing music, rescuing abused children or abandoned animals, or building homes for the needy. It's using any heart-and-soul–centered ritual, which for some is most helpful in the form of prayer, while others use meditation. Again, it's different things for different people, but it is always good for what ails you.

I recently treated a woman with serious joint pain, and I asked her to talk to me about spirituality as she lives and feels it. Sue responded with, "I'm not religious. I leave that to my husband." I asked her where she felt energized and at peace and she said, "When I'm in my garden." A backyard garden is as true a spiritual locus as a church or temple. It just needs to be identified so that you can call on it when you need it.

There was a study done by Jared Kass, PhD, and Lynn Cass, MA, that showed four different domains for spirituality. They found that people can experience spirituality:

- In their relationships with other people

- Within themselves

- Within nature

- Within a religion and a relationship with God

Like Sue, people typically do not fall into only one spiritual category. Also like Sue, many people confuse spirituality and religion. There's a significant difference between the two. Religion is more structured, with scriptures, rituals, and a day of worship. It is a cognitive code of beliefs in which you need to learn the customs, thinking, and behaviors of a God-centered system and internalize them. Oddly enough, I've met some people who are religious and follow the rules, but who are not necessarily spiritual.

I've found that some people have lost touch with their spirituality, or they feel life or pain has taken it from them.

We've become a goal-directed society, and while that's good, we bemoan a certain lack of accompanying inner satisfaction. "Is That All There Is?" can become a common theme song, even among highly successful men and women. Meanwhile, we live in a fairly high-pressure society, and we inevitably encounter negative stress and anxiety, which can help create, as Paul Tillich called it in *The*

Courage to Be, a kind of spiritual "insecurity." When you are over-come by stress and anxiety, you can have the perception that "life lacks fundamental meaning and that no God or Ground of Being exists." This perception may lead to a vicious circle. You're stressed and anxious, you feel spiritual doubt, and then, because you feel that life lacks meaning and that there is no higher power, you feel more stressed and anxious.

So while we work and aspire for more, meet obligations, raise families, and earn a living, seeing life as only a series of goals replaced by other, newer goals is usually not enough. It is spirituality that contributes the soul to any relationship, enterprise, or healing process.

Because spirituality is so important, I've put together a few of the components that you can examine for yourself. The journey of being healed is always a personal one—healing is hard work, and no one can do it for you. But you can do it for yourself!

What Spirituality Does for Healing: The Religious View

Spirituality is, paradoxically, spontaneously natural. It is as much about loving nature and feeling that "lift" as it is about finding comfort in the rituals of religion. When spirituality is focused on a belief in the unknown and the unseen, and an acceptance and a trust in God, it usually involves following a religion. Incidentally, God is not always part of the religious or spiritual process. Buddhists, for example, don't believe in a God so much as in a higher power or in enlightenment and knowledge. Buddhists' spirituality comes from a sense of their connectedness to something larger than themselves.

For others, a belief in God is enough, and they follow no religion.

Those qualities of intangibility and invisibility about God can make the concept of spirituality more difficult to grasp when you strive to understand it and summon comfort from it. But when you do connect to it deeply, you may be able to endure anything.

Landis Vance, a gifted hospital chaplain at a Washington, D.C., clinic and a good friend, deals with patients' physical and spiritual suffering every day. Landis had an interesting career, starting out as a banker. Many years ago, she was very ill, and as she says, she "came out the other end of it completely different and wanting to change my life." When one of her doctors suggested that she should be a hospital chaplain, she explored the idea in depth and found it was her calling.

In this role, she hears the most intimate feelings that patients would not otherwise divulge. Landis explains: "Some people are very angry about having a disorder and being in pain, and they're mad at God but won't acknowledge it. They think if God loved them, they would be okay. One patient I worked with was raised in a strict evangelical Christian tradition and feared revealing her anger with God at church or to her family. Allison felt she'd lost all faith because now, hurting so badly, she believed God wasn't trustworthy."

How difficult it is for people who are devout to suddenly doubt their faith and, at the same time, deal with physical pain! How does such a person find some resolution? As a chaplain, the first step Landis takes is to give such people permission to voice their fears and doubts. "I help them identify that they're mad at God in any way they want. Then I ask them to look back and see how God *had* acted positively in their lives. With Allison, it was an important exercise. She discovered that she didn't have faith in God because she'd been told to, but because she felt she knew who God is for her, and that God *was* trustworthy. That revelation gave her comfort, and she could talk about how angry she was about being in pain while reconnecting to her spiritual life."

One of the tools that I believe in when counseling someone dealing with chronic pain—and one that Landis uses, too—is a "spiritual assessment," which asks patients to answer questions about these very personal feelings. There are a number of standardized assessments with slightly different approaches, but all of them reveal your "spiritual landscape." For instance, one test focuses on the importance of a person's faith to them, whether they participate in a religious community, how they want a doctor to address or not address faith in their medical treatment, and even whether they can see the future in a positive way.

There are other points that you are asked to consider in this test that deal specifically with religious issues, such as your image of God—and not everyone has one. It also asks if you believe in a personal God and if you believe that God is a punishing God or that God gave you this pain to punish you.

How does this reflect on coping with pain? There has been a lot of research on positive and negative religious coping and, among the results, it was found that if people believe that God is wrathful, they are more likely to be sicker and more likely to die of their disease than if they think God is loving. Other studies have looked at prayer and whether or not people believe their prayers will be answered. Overall, big studies show that people with a high degree of spiritual well-being report a higher quality of life even if they have a higher level of pain.

Basically, everyone agrees that regardless of your religious orientation, the purpose and meaning you give to your life are very much connected to your spirituality, and these tests help us see how.

What's important is that it's possible to help people who, like Allison, may temporarily doubt their faith or believe God is punishing them—without changing their religious beliefs. As you know, some people believe that pain and disease are a punishment from God or that they didn't pray "right." Counseling from someone like Landis, who is a chaplain, or an empathetic psychotherapist, or the very doctor who is treating you can bring relief. The key is for you to understand what your ethnic and religious traditions mean to you and how you connect to them, and then decide if you are able to find comfort and emotional sustenance in them. When you fully understand how you connect to your religious traditions, you can effectively pick and choose what you hold on to for strength. With the help of spiritual counselors, you will learn to identify the positive, potentially healing aspects of your spirituality.

Patients have often told me that having chronic pain strengthened their spirituality and faith because the illness provided them with a wakeup call. That's pretty positive! So, if spirituality is sustaining and enlightening, can it also give rise to optimism? Landis says, "I think spirituality has a lot to do with optimism—not just optimism in general, but when you have to dig down deep, like when you're having chronic pain, and you know it's not a character trait but a part of your spirituality. Secondly, optimism depends on the religious framework people are in. One of the most frequent beliefs you hear from patients is that 'God does everything for a reason.' I also hear, 'God doesn't give you any more than you can handle'—another hopeful statement in the middle of a crisis. And whether you agree with either belief or not, it's a way of trying to cope. What comes out is a belief in a loving God and that everything will be okay."

To really cope, you need to have an "adult faith" to sustain you. "Many of the people I see," Landis says, "are those whose religious and spiritual formation tended to stop at adolescence. Parents pay attention to a child's spiritual growth until the child is about 13 or 14, unless the child continues on with religious services or schools."

Since many people today have the faith structures and systems of someone who is in junior high school, when a life-threatening illness occurs, they don't have an adult faith that can stand up to the challenge. Their spirit doesn't have the ability to incorporate all that suffering because they're still bound by their childhood beliefs. "A lot of what we do as spiritual counselors," Landis adds, "is help people grow into an adult faith that can handle the vicissitudes of life."

It's true that spiritual concerns are the most overlooked aspect of pain management, but hopefully that won't be the case for much longer. Whether it's our interconnectedness with others, nature, and the transcendent or the struggle to reconcile our beliefs of how the world "should" work with our actual experiences in life, it's time to change—and expand our spiritual universe.

Spiritual Assessment

I want to fill you in on the kinds of questions you'll find on spiritual assessment tests and why I believe they're important for you, your doctor, and your caregiver. Simply, by your answers, you can evaluate how you're coping with your illness and dealing with pain.

The tests perform a vital function by providing information about how you're coping spiritually and emotionally. Your answers are useful for doctors like me who can speak directly to such personal matters, for those who are more comfortable distancing themselves from their patients' feelings, and for those who worry about offering unrealistic reassurances.

A team of doctors/researchers looked at this very point in an article in *The Oncologist*. They found that caregivers tend to feel that "strong emotions such as guilt, anger, or anxiety will be unleashed by broaching the question of spirituality, and they might be unable to deal with those emotions." Thus, practitioners worry about handling your feelings and your story with sensitivity. Furthermore, the article continues, some doctors fear they'll be blamed for upsetting a patient by bringing up spiritual issues, while others fear that such a discussion will bring them too close to a patient, and they'll be badly hurt if the patient dies. Ultimately, the study concluded that for the doctor, "the courage required to confront such fears itself renews one's conviction that this is an important and rewarding aspect of clinical care." Questionnaires can really help doctors broach the topic.

As good as your doctor may be, she may not be able to help you with matters of spirituality to the extent that a spiritual advisor can. I feel safe in saying that any spiritual advisor who works at a hospital will have access to a number of questionnaires that will help you figure out where you are spiritually.

If you want to examine your spirituality, you can ask your doctor to direct you to a spiritual advisor and ask to be given the questionnaires. These questionnaires have been formatted so that it is easy for you to answer the questions. They're set up so that the questions are sensitive to cultural, religious, racial, gender, and ethnic differences.

There are a number of questionnaires that are commonly used for research and clinical purposes. One is called "The Inventory of Positive Psychological Attitudes," and it measures a resilient worldview. Another is "The Confidence in Life and Self" questionnaire, which looks at how people buffer stress and facilitate the prevention of stress-related psychological and physical disorders. A third questionnaire is "The Index of Core Spiritual Experiences (INSPIRIT)," which also measures the elements of spirituality that contribute to the formation of a resilient worldview but does not measure spiritual well-being.

Your Spirituality

I've put together a list of questions adapted from questionnaires I use at the hospital. My questionnaire is meant to help you clarify how you feel spiritually and how you use those feelings to help healing. Of course, there are no right or wrong answers to *any* questions about spirituality—what you feel and believe is entirely subjective, personal, and valid. Think about your answers and write them down. If you have no answer to a question the first time around, get back to it when you can.

• Do you consider yourself to be spiritual or religious?

_____

_____

• Would you say that you're (circle one):

(a) very spiritual or religious

(b) somewhat spiritual or religious

(c) not very spiritual or religious

• Do you believe in the higher power we call God?

_____

_____

• How does your image or definition of God make you feel?

_____

_____

• Did you ever have an intense spiritual experience that gave you:

☐ A feeling of profound inner peace

☐ A feeling of joy or ecstasy

☐ A feeling of intense belonging

☐ A feeling of overwhelming love

☐ A feeling that you'd just experienced God's presence

☐ A feeling of acceptance or forgiveness

• What importance does faith or belief have in your life?

_____

_____

• How often do you use your time for spiritual or religious thoughts or practices? (Circle one.)

(a) From once a day to a few times a day, every day

(b) From once a week to once a month

(c) From once every few months to once a year

(d) Rarely or never

• Are you part of a spiritual or religious community?

_____

• How do you participate in this group or community?

_____

_____

- What is your role?

_____

_____

- In what ways is this group a source of support for you?

_____

_____

- Are there any spiritual or secular symbols related to this religious community's beliefs that are significant for you? Why?

_____

_____

- Were there any religious or spiritual rituals in your home as a child?

_____

_____

- Have you carried on observing them? If so, why? If not, why not?

_____

_____

- Do you feel a sense of real thankfulness for your life, no matter what?

_____

_____

- Would you say that your illness has strengthened your spiritual beliefs?

_____

_____

- Have your beliefs influenced how you've taken care of yourself in this illness?

_____

_____

- Do you believe that whatever happens with your illness, things will be okay?

_____

_____

- Do you worry about dying?

_____

_____

- Do you feel you have a reason for living? How would you describe it?

_____

_____

- Do you think your life has been productive?

_____

_____

• Do you have a sense of meaning and purpose?

_____

_____

• Can you reach deep inside yourself for comfort?

_____

_____

• Do you feel loved?

_____

_____

• Do you feel love and compassion for others?

_____

_____

• If there are any spiritual gaps in your life, would you say it is because:

☐ You have little or no sense of harmony within yourself

☐ Your sense of harmony has been replaced with feelings of confusion, exhaustion, anxiety, and anger

☐ You have trouble feeling any peace of mind

☐ Your illness has made you doubt your ability to cope

☐ You feel anger toward a higher power or God for allowing this illness

☐ You fear that a higher power or God has abandoned you

☐ You believe you cannot forgive yourself for what you've done wrong

☐ You believe you cannot forgive others who have hurt you

☐ You are unsure if your life is part of a large spiritual force

• In looking back at and thinking about your answers to the above questions, to what extent would you say that spirituality plays an important part in understanding or coping with life?

_____

_____

• Are there specific elements of medical care that your religion discourages or forbids? To what extent have you followed these guidelines?

_____

_____

• What spiritual or religious knowledge or understanding would strengthen the relationship between you and your doctor?

_____

_____

• Are there barriers to the relationship between you and your doctor based on religious or spiritual issues?

_____

_____

I bet you'll know a lot more about yourself spiritually after you've answered these questions.

The Medical View

Let's go directly into the doctor's office and start with taking a patient's history. Doctors have to listen for what's really going on, since patients can answer questions with asides and digressions along with medical information. Ask a patient how they're feeling, and we could hear something like, "I get home from work and lie down on the couch. My husband sees me and makes jokes about how lazy I am," or "The migraine was so bad, I kept making mistakes at a meeting with a client." Doctors often disregard these bits of information, even though they may contain revealing messages about patients' fears and suffering. Doctors traditionally attend to the body rather than the spirit and either fail to diagnose suffering or disregard it as less important than diagnostic information.

Until recently, suffering was not considered, never mind routinely listed, as a potential complication on a patient's record. People, remember, suffer not only from physical pain or other aspects of disease but in some cases from its treatment as well. In fact, in a multinational survey, physical pain was listed as the least frequent cause of suffering. Rather, the more common reasons were distress at being a burden to others or having some discomfort other than pain. Such discomfort may be caused by marital problems or dealing with losses, such as people leaving; not getting the job you want; losing the job you have; getting older; or losing certain abilities, such as being able to drive. Discomfort may also arise from moving into an assisted-living facility or from a sense that you haven't accomplished your goals in life.

Happily, attention to spirituality is making a difference in medical care.

Science has already found real connections between negative emotions, such as anxiety and depression, and many physical illnesses, such as high blood pressure and chronic back pain. Similarly, researchers are now more closely examining the biological connections to spirituality. A good case can be made for the positive impact spirituality has on alleviating stress and pain.

In the journal *Family Medicine* researchers stated that the significant correlation between a patient's health and spirituality is a "new frontier in medicine." I'll stand up and cheer for that! Patients have indicated their desire for doctors to address spirituality as well as attend to their medical problems, and for good reason: Patients whose doctors *did* address spirituality had significant positive differences in both overall health and physical pain.

There's a lot of traveling in this new frontier.

One stop was made by researchers who concluded that core spiritual experiences may be a natural capacity of the human organism and that this "potential resource should be studied more fully." Other studies are following core spiritual experiences, including laughter and an attachment to pets (remember Debbie's pal, Lola the chicken?) and how each contributes to positive psychological attitudes. In fact, observations show that core spiritual experiences may very well contribute to a reduction in medical symptoms and to an improved quality of life.

How does spirituality make a difference in alleviating pain during a difficult illness like cancer? From both personal and professional experience, I know that a cancer diagnosis significantly contributes to emotional distress, a sense of panic, and confusion. Then there is the cancer pain itself, resulting from tumor involvement or side effects of treatments, which also may have a tremendous impact on your thoughts and attitudes.

Doctors writing in *Cancer Practice*, in a study titled "An Integrated Psychosocial-Spiritual Model for Cancer Pain Management," agreed that unrelieved cancer pain can result in lowered self-esteem, self-defeating thoughts, a pessimistic attitude, and catastrophic thinking. "Individuals also create meaning of their pain," the authors say, "especially in times of significant pain flare-ups and stress from the anticipation of pain." So, if you have cancer, and you feel pain anywhere in your body, you believe that this pain signifies a turn for the worse. You give this pain the meaning that you will soon die. If you have rheumatoid arthritis and wake up with increased pain, you associate it with becoming disabled and needing to get around in a wheelchair. The authors concluded, though, that it is very important for a medical team to have full knowledge of how the patient's beliefs and perceptions contribute to pain issues. "A thorough spiritual assessment, accompanied by ongoing spiritual care, implemented at time of diagnosis," they say, "could minimize much of the pain and suffering that patients experience while living and dying with cancer."

Yet another study, called "When the Spirit Hurts," took a very forward-thinking approach and found that while doctors may not be able to alleviate suffering in the same manner or to the same degree as they can physical pain, the simple recognition that a patient is suffering "is the first step in a truly holistic approach, allowing the patient to feel the therapeutic power of compassion and begin healing." I can only agree with the researchers who concluded that "ultimately, the most effective treatment of the whole person cannot occur unless we address concurrent suffering."

Spirituality definitely provides an interpretive framework for many patients in handling illness. To me, this new journey is worth taking.

A Personal View

I've always felt that it was important to connect to the spirit of a patient by showing interest and compassion and demonstrating a joy for life. It makes a real difference in how patients feel. I'm even willing to add a little showmanship. If it's Mardi Gras, I'll roam the halls of my hospital in a getup—even a coconut bra and grass skirt; on St. Patrick's Day, I've tinted a very willing patient's hair bright green. And in general, I'll push my teacart festooned with floppy hats and feather boas, from which I'm happy to serve high tea to patients who have lost their hair to chemo. Strange as my approach may seem to many, it works! Is getting a few laughs while in costume about spirituality? Of course.

I've always been a spiritual person who is also religiously observant. I've spent many years specializing in treating people in pain, and I still think about how to improve the level of healing and feeling spiritually intact for my patients. The journey of being healed is always a personal one and is always hard work, and no one can do it for you. I learned this as a patient, not just as a doctor.

Like everyone, I've asked myself, "Why do people die and what, truly, is the meaning of life?" My father told me "life" was about family, work, and relationships. For me, that philosophy was never stronger than when I was diagnosed with breast cancer. The diagnosis made me face my own mortality. At that point, you first think you'll never know joy again, or give joy to others, or live out your aspirations. When I calmed down a bit, I knew the diagnosis would give me a second chance to reexamine priorities and explore what I felt about "meaning" and values.

The meaning of my life was immediately clear to me: I wanted to see my children grown up, married, and happy in their own choices. Working with patients who are very ill has also played an important part in having a meaning for being. Reaching out and helping others is very healing. Sitting by the bedside daily with people who are ill helps me feel the presence of the light every day. This is a true gift.

I received my diagnosis just 6 weeks before I was to begin my job in Bethesda. At that time, I was on top of the world. Nearly 250 of my peers competed to get the position I would soon hold—a post that offered a chance to take the nascent field of palliative care out of the oncology wards and hospices and use those techniques in the nation's premier research hospital. Through it, I could help advance both the science of palliative care and its credibility in the medical community.

It was Christmas 1999, and I was trying to decide how to tell my bosses in Camden that I was leaving. I went for my annual mammogram at the hospital radiology lab and thought little of it. Then the technician jolted me out of my reverie when he asked to take another image, followed by the words every woman dreads: "I think we have a problem here." He ordered a biopsy. I was numb as I walked from the radiology lab directly to the office Christmas party under way in the next office. A knot the size of a boulder filled my chest while I tried to carry on with holiday cheer. Inside, I was counting off what was possibly next: surgery, chemo, radiation, or even more dire outcomes at this crucial moment in my life.

The news was bad: The biopsy showed cancer. I elected for a double mastectomy, and I scheduled the surgery for just after the holidays. I knew that a double mastectomy was aggressive therapy for my condition, but it offered the best chance of never having to face breast cancer again. My family and I were making peace with the decision when we all started off on our New Year's holiday in Pennsylvania.

I had never wanted the comfort of intimate surroundings more than I did that tumultuous year, and Lancaster fulfilled the need. We'd spent many New Years in a charming old hotel right in the middle of Amish country. We love the town's pretzel factory and the lake behind the hotel, where the management maintains a flock of ducks the guests can feed with bread sold lakeside. On New Year's Eve, everything was just as we expected it. The kids splashed around in the indoor swimming pool, we watched the ball drop on a television feed from Times Square, and within an hour, all of us were packed off to bed. After a day of all the soothing, familiar activities, I was feeling relaxed and positive. I was anticipating a successful surgery and the beginning of a wonderful new job with my cancer in remission.

I woke up during the night with a stabbing pain in my back so severe that it immobilized me. My anxiety immediately magnified that pain from a 5 to a 10. As an oncologist, my thoughts instantly associated my symptoms with the worst possible outcome. "I know what this is," I thought. "The cancer spread from my breast to my spine! This is metastatic cancer, and I am going to die from it."

After my hysterical self-diagnosis, my thoughts for the next 24 hours were all about my children. How would they get on without me? I knew they were resourceful and survivors and, like me, would take life as it came and figure out how to cope. I also knew they couldn't have a more loving and stable father than my husband, Carl. But I wanted to live. I bargained with God. Okay, let me live at least long enough to be at my son, Stephen's, bar mitzvah that coming spring and, if I could manage to eke out more time, attend my daughter, Rebecca's, bat mitzvah 3 years later. If I could see my children get to college and then stand alongside them under the wedding canopy, those extra years would be lovely bonuses. Beyond that, everything else was gravy, as far as I was concerned. But if all the life I was allowed was 3 more years and simple celebration of my kids' maturity at 13, I would savor my luck every day.

I got back to work on January 2, and the doctors determined that my back pain was from a herniated disk. My perception of the meaning of my pain quickly dropped from a 10 to an 8. Did the pain diminish during x-ray? Not very likely. One thing I know: By the time I picked up my steroid prescriptions, it had dropped to a 6. I truly believe the pain ebbed because its meaning had changed. It was not the pain that would define my last days. The pain wouldn't kill me. I put pain in its place!

My bargaining with God to give me just a few more years with my children made the link between me and my patients even stronger than it had been before. I understood how they felt and why they were willing to endure painful treatments just to get a few more days with those they loved. That said, what did I truly value? The career could go, the face and body, too. Prestige and possessions never mattered much to me. I thought back to when I was growing up, when as a teenager, I became religious, unlike my family. Back then, I was looking for an answer that had less to do with the activities of this world and more to do with the promise of the next. When I got sick with cancer, I finally understood what my father meant when he said life is about family, work, and relationships. Every step I took toward healing was a step deeper into what I felt were spiritual values.

I went to work every day, although my staff and family protested that I needed to rest. I wanted to remain useful. I not only took medication, I turned to a few complementary and experimental treatments for my back pain. Every day, I wore a brace with magnets in it, and I kept applying a heating pad. I took breaks for therapeutic baths and acupuncture treatments. By the end of the day, I was beat. I could barely eat dinner and say good night before going straight to bed.

Healing Pain

But for me, contact with my patients made the pain manageable. As the weeks went on, I had a greater appreciation for the astonishing efforts they made despite their physical conditions. I saw how they strived to settle issues with estranged family, to give what they could, and to remain active—in fact, to live with vigor and purpose even with chronic pain. My interactions with them also made me aware of the areas in my life that I needed to heal.

Although I tell my patients that illness is a chance to stop and smell the roses, months of my life had gone by in a blink without my taking my own advice. I became obsessed with work, being around people, interacting—proof that I was alive and capable. I forgot about savoring the smell of a fresh peach, watching the sunlight in my backyard as it faded over the trees at sunset, and being soothed by the wind chimes at my bedroom window. My family makes a point of eating dinner together every night, but then, my mind was on other matters and I was missing. Finally, I pulled out of the trance. Although it was difficult for me to eat during my illness, I sat at the table with the kids, cherishing their facial expressions, their clever ideas, even their disputes. These small, sweet delights were always available to me, but I had zipped along taking them for granted. My illness gave them all back to me: the things that give life meaning.

Of course, I don't claim to have found the meaning of life. That is an issue both too personal and too general for any one individual to respond to. At the onset of illness, though, this concept becomes more intimate and specific. You jump from "What is the meaning of life" to "What is the meaning of *my* life? What gives *my* life meaning, and how can I give it more?"

No one knows what enriches your spirit like you do. Please act on it now.

Helping Yourself: Four Ideas to Take with You on the Road to Healing

Spirituality is a multifaceted concept in which one size does not fit all. While there really isn't any formula for finding or enhancing your own spirituality, there are four "keys" that are irrevocably connected to using spirituality to help healing.

Key #1: Empty yourself of your burdens. Doing so gets you through pain and helps break the logjam of confused feelings. This involves giving up control of the things you can't control, accepting things you cannot change, and moving on. It involves reorienting how you think about life. It's not easy, and you have to be brutally honest with yourself about what self-sabotaging attitudes you live by, what you're holding on to from the past, why you're holding on to it, and why you need to let it go if it is still hurting you!

Dan is a good example of this. A man in his late thirties, Dan came to see me because of pain due to an abdominal malignancy. Prior to his illness, he'd been working as a psychologist, but since his diagnosis, he had given up his practice and stopped working. Dan's issue? He was waiting for the next shoe to drop. He was panicked about lack of control over his disease, he feared a recurrence, and he doubted that he could heal. He became paralyzed as a functioning person. He was alive but not truly living.

When I talked to him about this, he said, "I've put my life on hold for the past 11 months." We spoke about why he needed to let go of his feelings about that lack of control. I explained that we would need to "reframe" his thinking so he could begin to live again by accepting life as it is. For example, it was important for Dan to reconnect with what he could do—be a capable psychotherapist—and *do it*, rather than focus on what he feared he would not be able to do if his illness got worse. By the end of the interview, Dan agreed to plan a trip with his wife and try going to a religious service, though he wasn't sure there was a greater being. Even though he wasn't sure about God, it helped him to realize that his life was a part of a greater community.

Key #2: Remember that healing is a personal journey that no one can make for you. Healing is hard work, and it's different for everyone—but every person in pain can seek help and ask for it anywhere. For many people, help is asking for healing through prayer. For others, life's creative activities—like music, art, dance, a connection to nature, cooking, caring for others, humor, massage, or spiritually based disciplines like Reiki or tai chi—help healing. Use all your senses of hearing, smell, touch, taste, and sight to be in the moment and intensify the experience. It will bring you peace and a sense of being centered.

Key #3: Don't be afraid to let things go. When one door closes, another always opens. You may find forgiveness and be able to express gratitude, which is so important in healing.

A patient of mine, who recently died, had been struggling with lung cancer. Pete had been divorced for many years and had a grown son and daughter who were married and living in other states. Pete was in his late fifties and lived with a young girlfriend in her early twenties at the time of his diagnosis. When his illness became terminal, he realized that he'd sacrificed important relationships with his children and wanted to have them in his life until the end. He also knew in his heart that the tempestuous relationship with his girlfriend was not where he wanted to be, and they split up.

Pete spent months redeveloping new, healthy relationships with his ex-wife and children. In closing the door to his life with his girlfriend, he opened opportunities he never thought he would have with family he'd always loved. As a result of this, Pete lived and died in peace, feeling healed and whole.

Key #4: Keep in mind that there is no magic gift box with your name on it, holding everything you ever wanted. A good, pain-free, and spiritual life cannot be handed to you as a gift. Finding the meaning of your life is possible only by looking within and examining yourself and your own beliefs. Your inner strength and the answers to your questions are deep within your soul. The closest you can get to a magic box is one that, when opened, reveals a mirror into which you can look as deeply as you like.

Most of all, you'll get the gift of knowing that spirituality is both transforming and restorative.

CHAPTER 5

"Keep Your Fork!"

Develop Your Appetite for Optimism

I know an astonishing woman whose passion for life does not wane, no matter how bad the news from her doctors. Jane faces the spread of cancer and increasing chronic pain on a daily basis in an inspiring, humor-filled, and relentlessly hopeful way. She has metastatic breast cancer, which for her means it has spread to her brain, lungs, and spinal cord, producing numerous life-threatening tumors. Seven years after her diagnosis, Jane believes in life with an unshakeable faith, and she thinks of herself as an optimist.

Although her condition is extreme, Jane so moves me that I hope she'll be an inspiring model for you as you adopt and live with a positive, life-affirming attitude. When you do, I know it will make coping with, accepting, and ultimately healing illness and pain more of a possibility. In fact, Jane's story is the inspiration for this chapter. She would be the first person to agree that negativity is life draining, period! Let me tell you her story by beginning with an excerpt from one of her e-mails to me.

"The doctor tells me I'm dying and wasn't going to treat me any more. But I'm not going anyplace soon. I refuse to accept what he said, and I went for a 13½-dose program of radiation for spinal cord tumors, which has restored the function of my left leg. I'll be around . . ."

Jane is the daughter of a man I treated for a chronic pain condition early on in my career. More than a decade after her father's treatment, Jane developed breast cancer. She tracked me down across the country and told me how my care had been important to her father, which meant a lot to me. It was, coincidentally, a momentous time for Jane to find me with the specific request that I help her plan her cancer treatment. I was addressing my own bout with the same disease at the same time. When I told her about my condition, we became an e-mail support system for each other. We also exchanged little gifts and tokens of encouragement that always arrived just when we needed that extra push.

As my condition improved, Jane's continued to worsen. Doctors were always giving her 6 months, or 2 months, or even a few weeks to live, yet she always beat their dire predictions while maintaining her droll, gallows sense of humor. During chemo, for example, she posted a picture of herself on her Web site captioned: "Bald in the USA." Through all this, she talked candidly about her condition to me, expressed hope for herself, and always ended her e-mails with the enigmatically silly "Keep your fork!"

After months of seeing this closing comment, I finally asked Jane what significance this had for her, and what it could mean to me. She was delighted to explain. Oddly enough, I received an answer to my question right before I was to lead a healing service at my temple. This was close on the heels of the catastrophic events of September 11, 2001. As the family was getting ready to leave home, my husband, Carl, brought in the mail. In the heaps of correspondence was a little package from Jane, along with this story.

A dying young woman received a final call from her pastor. As the visit came to a close, she told him she had one last wish— to be buried with a fork. When the pastor questioned her about this curious request, she told him this: In all her years of attending dinner parties, a certain ritual always occurred. As the main course was being cleared away, the hostess usually advised the guests to keep their forks. This meant that something wonderful was on the way, as yet unknown, such as a velvety chocolate mousse. Therefore, she confirmed to the pastor, she wanted to be buried with a fork because she was certain there would be something sweet, surprising, and blissful ahead for her.

The simple tale touched me deeply, especially when I unwrapped the accompanying silver fork that Jane had enclosed in the package. After all we'd been through together, her story of hope coming at this difficult time brought tears to my eyes. I talked about Jane at the healing service that night and spread her message: *Keep your fork!* Something good is on the way now.

Jane's fork has a place of honor on my teacart.

When people ask me what qualities Jane has to keep up that spirit, I say it is a combination of a love of life and an ability to not let physical and emotional pain take over. In all our years of correspondence and talks, I know that Jane has struggled with the same life issues that any of us would experience. Love and loss, success and failure, betrayal and trust, fear and courage, joy and misery, and so on. What makes her so life affirming is that she never allows negative feelings to take over. She's faced her demons, dealt with anger, and grieved over losses as we all do, on a daily basis. But Jane doesn't dwell on what's wrong and what's bad. She'd rather put her energy into healing, into connecting positively with the world—her form of spirituality—not into grieving over what cannot be changed.

I have another friend who also went through a few difficult years battling breast cancer, with a very similar attitude. Sybil told me that when she got her diagnosis, she went for a manicure and spent the rest of the day in denial. Then she spent half the next day in a panic. On the third day, she walked into an oncology ward, preparing for her first chemo treatment preceding surgery. She says, "I suddenly felt calm, but I was sure my mood would change, and fear and panic would set in. I decided that adding to the anxiety was pointless. Instead, I promised myself to spend no more than 10 minutes every morning on feeling sorry for myself and to stop myself from any negative thoughts after that. If ever I knew that life is too short, it was then."

Letting Go of Past Hurts

I know there are times when chronic pain is either so distracting or so severe that you cannot think about anything but wanting relief.

But I also know that holding on to negative attitudes and experiences from the past—what I call burdens—ultimately cannot help healing. In *The Power of Myth*, Joseph Campbell wrote that people say they're all seeking the meaning of life. "I don't think that's what we're really seeking," he said. "I think what we're seeking is an experience of being alive . . . of the *rapture* of being alive." This is what both Jane and Sybil have tapped into, each in her own way, and what I hope you can feel, too.

So while there is spiritual healing and spiritual power, there is also emotional healing and psychological power. This is, in some measure, gained by letting go of past hurts and defusing some of the incidents in your life that still trigger anger, fear, trepidation, or a need for an emotion-numbing drug (pharmaceuticals, street drugs, sugar, alcohol) and add to your physical pain. This "letting go" may be complicated, but I hope you'll at least think about freeing yourself from past problems. They're over with, and you cannot change what has happened.

What you can change is how you respond, and this is where your power lies.

Understanding Your Burdens

Burdens come in numerous forms, but what they have in common is how they prevent you from achieving peace, acceptance, and movement toward healing. Burdens can stem from many types of circumstances: an onerous childhood, an abusive parent, a brutal incident foisted upon you, failure to achieve a dream in school or on a job, a relationship with a generally difficult or nongiving partner, tragic loss, or the diagnosis of a disorder or disease. While the actual incident has long passed, you still feel the aftershock of the trauma as if it had happened yesterday. Those aftershocks can intensify whatever pain you feel from a physical condition.

Other burdens are self-imposed and are just as able to affect your pain level and how you cope with it. For example, many people are overly ambitious about meeting goals at a time when such goals make little sense. The pressure they put on themselves is physically debilitating and pain inducing. Here's what I mean: One of my patients, who had just remarried in her early fifties, bought a big house. She dreamed of it being a gathering place that would always smell like warm cookies and pot roast. Della and her husband, Scott, who was in his late fifties when they bought their huge home, were preparing for a future that included having their children from their previous marriages and their grandchildren visit frequently. Then Della was diagnosed with fibromyalgia.

To maintain the house, Della and Scott worked longer hours at stressful jobs that left them both cranky and depleted. Della's condition worsened. The house was a burden, and like most burdens, it was hurtful, despite the couple's good intentions. It took nearly a year for them to realize that their obsession with the place was harming them. The image of the "big, happy family home" had become too much a part of their identity and hope for the future. Della told me, "It is difficult to imagine a meaningful life without the big house to set the stage. We both wanted to make up to our kids what we didn't give them the first time around."

How she and her husband shortchanged themselves by believing that what they had done for their kids was lacking! Their kids went through demanding, "why can't we have this?" teenage years but grew up into otherwise loving children. Della's first marriage was a disaster. She got married too young, and her husband didn't want kids, so he pretty much neglected their girls. Scott's wife died in a car accident when his kids were both under 10 years old, and he always felt they lost out at having more "homey stuff they'd have with a mother."

In treating Della for her fibromyalgia, I also recommended counseling for her and for Scott. She and her husband shared a kind of burden of guilt about not having been good enough parents when, in fact, they *were*. They had good relationships with their children. Eventually, they realized that the extended family would be better served by selling the big house and scaling down. They bought a smaller house, and Della was able to change jobs and work only 3 days a week, giving her psychological and physical time to heal. "Now we can only accommodate one of our kids and the grandkids at a time, but that's okay. It's just as meaningful to us."

People are shaped by the burdens they carry as much as they are by their talents, disposition, spirituality, and goals. This is why it can be difficult to let go of these painful parts of your persona—they are literally part of you. It's never easy, but you owe yourself a chance to try. The relief that rushes in once a burden has been clarified and dropped from your way of life is significant.

Your Emotional State

To help you figure out what may be burdening you and affecting your pain level, answer these questions. Write down what you feel and go back to any question that you are unable to answer the first time around.

• Have you accepted your illness?

_____

_____

• Are you anxious?

_____

_____

• Are you sad?

_____

_____

• Do you feel angry or resentful that you have this pain?

_____

_____

- Do you feel lonely?

_____

_____

- Do you worry that your condition will get worse?

_____

_____

- Are you content with the present quality of your life?

_____

_____

- Do you have trouble feeling peace of mind?

_____

_____

- Can you comfort yourself?

_____

_____

- Do you think that whatever happens with your illness, things will be okay?

_____

_____

- Do you know you are lovable and that you do not have to make special efforts for others to be accepted and loved by them?

_____

_____

- Are you able to accept change in your life, or do you fight it to keep the status quo?

_____

_____

- Is your work fulfilling?

_____

_____

How You See Your Life Now
in Terms of Your Past

- Is there a single troubling milestone event that you believe shaped how you feel about yourself? What happened?

_____

_____

- Do you think this negative event still affects the decisions you make? If yes, how?

_____

_____

- Do you tend to replay negative or stressful events in your head over and over—even months or years after they happened?

_____

_____

- Do you feel that you have been taken advantage of by others in the past? Do you feel angry with yourself for not standing up to them better than you did?

_____

_____

- Do you feel that you never had the chance to achieve your best? If so, why do you believe that happened?

_____

_____

- Did you lose someone or something important to you when you were a child and still grieve the loss, or are you unable to grieve?

_____

_____

- Do you ever catch yourself being angry at or resentful of others, so much so that you feel it at the gut level?

_____

_____

• Do you ever catch yourself thinking in terms of "what's missing"?

_____

_____

Dropping Your Burdens: What You Need to Know to Let Them Go

As we all know, there's really no magical or easy way to release the burdens that you've carried with you over time. Yet, if you want to be free of what's causing you emotional setbacks, there's really only one thing to do: self-work. You'll need to answer the above questions honestly to best know yourself and work on defusing the problems. While awareness of what's hurting you is a serious step forward, it's not enough; enlightenment is never automatic. I've formulated a few steps for you to think about.

Give Yourself a Break

I've spoken to a number of psychologists, and they agree that the first step toward healing is to remove yourself from the victim role. Try not to reinforce the thinking that your burdens are worse than those of other people. As I explained earlier, there's no comforting answer to "Why me?" If you feel victimized by pain and painful events in your past, something's got to give. Even if it's true that your troubles are worse than those of others around you, the solution is to rise above dwelling in pain. Give up your burdens, not your energy for living with more joy.

A therapist I work with has noticed that some people at such a level of sadness or despair refuse counseling with a psychotherapist or psychiatrist. Some of these same people also will not join support groups. Support groups are targeted to people who have one specific health problem. They are usually run by a therapist, social worker, or medical doctor and can be found through a hospital or health organization. If you join a support group, you know that everyone there shares your problem, such as coping with chronic pain.

You can join a support group and also have psychotherapy sessions with a psychologist, psychoanalyst, or psychiatrist. These are accredited mental health practitioners, each with different levels of schooling and different degrees. A psychiatrist is a medical doctor who can also prescribe drugs. If you care to, you can have therapy one on one, find a therapist who specializes in family therapy (if that's your need), join a group that is run by the therapist or psychiatrist, or try all of these approaches.

The bottom line is that it's not a good idea to refuse help when you need it. There are many reasons why you might resist such help when you're in pain. Maybe it's because you don't want to hear about other people's pain. You fear that those stories will make you feel worse and as if you cannot do anything to help. Maybe you want others to listen to how pain is affecting you, but you feel embarrassed to talk in front of strangers. Or you fear that others won't have any sympathy for you.

Give yourself a break. If past burdens are still dragging you down, do everything you can to help yourself.

In my opinion, the 12-step programs, like Alcoholics Anonymous or Overeaters Anonymous, offer some of the best psychology when they suggest you ask yourself, "Do I have control over this?" If you don't, you can apply the philosophy of the group to learn to relinquish a victim stance and seek other ways of finding comfort and help. Many people have told me that the 12-step philosophy really makes sense in terms of dealing with chronic pain because it stresses taking responsibility for your actions and your life. If you think joining such a group will help you, give it a try. You can easily sit in on a meeting and see if any of the pointers or testimonials from attendees help you feel better. There are also many books on 12-step programs, so you can read about them first.

One of the truths of life is that not every problem will have a solution. The point is to find some productive way of resolving an issue even if you can't reconcile it. If nothing else, a resolution means that you have found a way to make your own peace, and that is most important in your healing process.

Grieve for Your Losses and Move On

We all talk about "what *was*": when it was "better," or when we were younger, or when we could run a marathon, or not worry about attracting the opposite sex, or get a good job that made us feel secure and accomplished. A part of growing older and maturing is to grieve for your youth, for past or lost opportunities, for those who have died—and for the wellness you once knew if you are in pain now.

Loss is part of life—there is no other way. But if you live for what was rather than for what *is* and what *will be*, you cannot fully heal or grow emotionally. Letting this burden go expands your universe. Psychoanalyst and theorist Erik Erikson called this task generativity, wherein you always have something to look forward to by operating from a future-oriented view of life. It is then that you can find things that give you pleasure at every stage of your life, and you learn to cope with loss.

Losses that have not been acknowledged, let alone grieved, are a pervasive block to healing and a major problem in our society. This was brought home to me, literally, in a dramatic way when I was talking to my son about the mandatory health course that he, as a high school junior, was required to take. The instructor spent less than 3 minutes on death and how it affects us as loss. This opened my eyes a lot.

Every day at work, I see how unacknowledged loss comes back to haunt my patients 100 percent of the time. I thought that I should do something about it and got together with a member of my staff. We devised a curriculum for teaching about loss and grief in a classroom at my son's school and were allowed to do it. Every single child in the class articulated at least one significant loss, and most had more than one. By the end of the first class, we discovered that more than *half* the students had strong unresolved feelings about their parents' divorces, deaths of loved ones, violent incidents from childhood, or sudden, job-related relocations across the country. This told me that easily more than 50 percent of these teenagers were holding in painful emotional experiences. Clearly, the other half of the students were taught by their families to cope with loss, whereas this half didn't have the benefit of such an education.

Which brings me to you. In the state of chronic pain, life's accumulated losses loom large. If you do not address them, grieve them, and accept how they have affected your life today, healing cannot move forward.

Forgive Yourself and Forgive Others

Forgiveness doesn't mean you have to forgive people just to be a good sport. I know it was a trend for a while for antagonists to face each other on a TV talk show, and for the person who'd been hurt to publicly forgive the person who had inflicted the pain. As a doctor specializing in healing pain, I know there's some sense in this theatrical display of the forgiveness game. A little forgiveness goes a long way. You don't have to forget, but do pardon yourself and others.

You may decide never to have contact, in any form, with the person who hurt you, and this is your choice. People get into trouble when they drag burdens down a lifelong destructive path. They use up energy and the best years of their lives by perpetuating the bad feelings associated with the offense. They stay angry instead of letting their burdens go with some form of palliative forgiveness.

Therefore, I suggest that you forgive yourself first. If you think you haven't done the best by yourself, know that you did what you could, as you could do it. Write it down, forgive yourself, then tear up the page.

Then forgive those who have hurt you. If you are unable to contact the person directly, or if the person is dead, write down what happened, when, and how you feel—then tear up the page!

Then ask others whom you hurt to forgive you. If you are unable to contact them, or if they're gone, follow the same procedure. Detail the situation that caused the rift between you, forgive yourself, and tear up the page.

Forgiveness brings with it a lightening of burdens. You're no longer a victim—in fact, you're not even a survivor, but a victor. Real acceptance of forgiveness results in an appreciation of life, the knowledge that you're willing to risk again and that you may be hurt again, but not devastated.

Most of all, I would like you to remember these critical points about forgiveness.

- Forgiveness allows you to resume your personal power. The grievance is no longer a barrier to healing or emotional growth.

- Although others may offer to intercede, thank them and say no. You can't do anyone's forgiveness work for them, and they cannot do it for you. For forgiveness to have a changing effect, it is important to take responsibility for the act.

- Do your utmost to understand that there may be no way to compensate you for a terrible wrong, such as an abusive childhood. All you can do is disengage from those responsible, let go, and move forward.

While love and empathy bind us to others in a blissful way, the stuff that creates burdens in life—rejection, abandonment, exploitation, and abuse—binds us to others in a pain-making way. One beneficial by-product of forgiveness is the chance to make changes in your perspective on others. Remember what Viktor Frankl and other psychologists tell us: We can't change what happened, but we *can* change how we respond. With a change of perspective, you can make emotionally based changes that put past burdens behind you. When you do, you can:

- Feel grateful that you've made it to this point and take responsibility for what comes next.

- Figure out the answer to the question, "What burdens are stopping me from healing, and how do I discharge them?"

- Trust in your courage to face what went wrong and make life better now. This courage provides emotional and spiritual ballast.

- Allow yourself to feel good again. With a release of burdens and forgiveness, you can reacquaint yourself with feeling pleasure, feeling for others, and connecting to your senses to feel alive.

Anger: Talking It Out or Letting It Out

I've mentioned anger in this chapter for a very good reason: Anger is one of those emotions that fuels and refuels itself. Anger creates bad stress, and as you know, bad stress affects the body adversely.

What makes another person angry may not bother you or me.

Some of the patients I see who tend to be the angriest live in an all-or-nothing state, and their feelings mimic it—they're "madly" in love, they're "terrified" that a teenage son will crash the car, they feel "broke" when there's money in the bank, or they'll "kill themselves" if the pain doesn't stop. Speaking about life in catastrophizing language is never more fraught with emotion than when pain frustrates them. As a person with head-splitting migraines and a back problem, I know what it's like to feel angry when the pain is relentless.

Where does the anger go? How can you deal with pain so that anger, too, does not become a burden?

Managing Anger

There have been entire books written about anger and whether venting or not venting can make you feel better. My sense is to get it out in a safe way and not to drop it on the first person who walks into the room or to make it your way of relating to the world. For some people, a health crisis brings out a lifetime of feeling anger, and after squelching it for so long, they vent in frustration, despair, and fear. A state of rage is not conducive to healing.

If you're angry, talk it out and get the rage out of your system as calmly as you can.

I recently treated a patient who had a very difficult life. Maya grew up in poverty, put herself through secretarial school, and got married to a man who, after a few years of marriage, left her to raise their daughter alone. At 45 years old, Maya had sickle cell disease, a chronic, life-threatening, and genetically inherited illness. Sickle cell patients have many special issues because of their disease, one of which is having several family members all suffering at the same time from the same chronic and painful illness.

Many people with sickle cell disease do not live as long as Maya has. The disease distorts hemoglobin cells that are normally round, making them crescent shaped. And since hemoglobin doesn't travel through the blood vessels the same way as normal cells, these patients end up having significant bone pain when they go into crisis. This crisis stage requires hospitalization for intravenous antibiotics, usually some oxygen, and intravenous pain medicines.

Maya lived with her sister and worked part-time because of her state of health. When she first came in to see me, she was angry about everything—about having the disease, about the hospital insurance system, and about the treatments. She was even angry with all doctors who had ever cared for her. She distrusted me. I learned that her 24-year-old daughter, who was pregnant, was a carrier of the disease, and her child would have it. About this Maya felt not only angry but also guilty.

In the past, Maya had bad experiences with doctors not believing the extent of her pain. I knew she wanted us to prove ourselves to her—that we believed her pain existed to the degree she said it did. When she checked into the hospital, Maya's anger took over. When she wanted more pain medication, she literally walked down the halls screaming at the top of her lungs. The nursing staff did not know what to do. I called an associate at our spiritual ministry to talk to her and help her to shift her attitudes and calm down. For this was the odd thing about Maya: When any one of us on her medical team asked her why she had so much rage, she would say, "Who's angry?" She did not recognize anger in herself. She did recognize that she had no trust in medicine or in doctors. My mission was to engage her confidence. If any woman needed to "keep her fork," it was Maya.

It took a while, but we finally connected with her in a positive and meaningful way. We adjusted her medication, and we found that Maya was willing to try alternate therapies, too, such as Reiki. It settled her down (Reiki is good for significantly decreasing anxiety), but what most changed her life was music therapy. She rediscovered a talent she had always had when she was growing up but never had the chance to express: singing. She's left us with affection and a CD she made of her favorite blues songs.

Maya is now on stable doses of methadone. She moved out of her sister's house and into a nursing home situation, which works out well for her. The nursing home provided her with five women friends who look out for each other—an important social network for her. When she left the hospital, we had a tea party for her and gave her a fork and her favorite hat to take to the home.

The Journal Approach

Everyone may be different in how they cope with anger, but what all people have in common is a need to talk about their specific experiences in some way. I know that many people are very private and don't like expressing anger in front of strangers, including doctors. If you feel you can share your feelings of anger with a loved one, friend, or someone on your medical team, do so. If not, try the journal approach. Get it all out on paper.

Beverly Kirkhart, author of *My Healing Companion*, describes journaling for anger management. Her book is a journal about fighting breast cancer, which came upon her around the time when her marriage broke up and she was bankrupt. Keeping a journal about having cancer "changed her life for the better."

Anger is a commonly felt emotion when you are diagnosed with a life-changing disorder that creates chronic pain or with a life-threatening disease, which you are struggling to fight and bearing the accompanying pain. "I'm an emotional time bomb," Kirkhart wrote. "I'm a pressure cooker ready to blow up! I resent what has happened to me. Or I hate feeling out of control." Are these healthy thoughts? Yes, but only because they are genuinely what she feels and needs to express. Holding in anger is far more destructive.

A journal like this provides a safe place to record your feelings, and Kirkhart had the right idea to begin healing her body and her soul. I want to encourage you to do the same: Write down a few phrases to describe how you feel, no matter how incendiary or irrational you think they are. Say what you need to say and get it out, once and for all. But above all, be kind to yourself. Your anger will diminish and be less destructive when you realize the pursuit of healing and health is much more motivating and powerful than anger.

If you don't want to tackle a journal, try writing a healing letter to yourself that describes your condition in terms of feelings. Does your condition bring up anger and resentment, fears of what will happen to you tomorrow, remorse and regrets? Write how you feel about the people you most care about. Include those for whom you feel love and appreciation, those you forgive, and those for whom you feel anger. Then think about those who are there for you with compassion and forgiveness and who appreciate you, and about those who are angry at you.

To do this exercise, make yourself comfortable and write until you feel you've exposed your emotions on paper. It may take several times to complete this process, but stay with it to reap the benefits. After you complete the letter, release your feelings with a burning ceremony. Throw the letter into a fireplace, bucket, or safe, fireproof receptacle and burn it! This will help you let go of the past and enable you to begin to accept your life as it is.

As an example, you could write:

- On anger: "I'm angry that I have fibromyalgia, and I feel that each new day means more pain and less of a good life."

- On fears: "I'm sad that my life may never be the same. Some days, I am afraid I will die in pain."

- On love, compassion, or appreciation: "I never could have gotten through this last year without my husband being there. I know how hard it was for him, and I appreciate everything he's done. I may have pain, but I appreciate life, the people I love, and what I have."

Operate from Strength

Even in a weakened state, people exhibit remarkable strengths.

I want to assure you that you can use those strengths to reclaim a healthy sense of self. Do everything you can to shift your attitude away from what you have lost to the aspects of your character that have survived and intensified as some of the busy work of life has receded. These new traits could be humor, clarity about what has real value to you, an understanding of what and whom you love—as well as to whom you want to express that love.

Tap Into What Gives Your Life Meaning

Distraction is an important element in managing chronic pain. Focus on the pleasures of life to reacquaint yourself with the power of the senses. Many times, it's hard to remember what it is about life you enjoy. Or if you do remember it, it is with a wistfulness that assumes you will never be able to know that contentment again. Perhaps you will no longer be able to ski down a steep run at your favorite resort, but most likely, you can bring some element of the sport back into your life. Don't cut out activities and interests from your life because your circumstances have changed. Read about them, watch videos about them, keep up with the news, and do it all without resentment.

Examine what you may be missing by having a pain condition, what you love, and what it is you have left undone. Nothing is as mood elevating as creating a plan for getting as many of these things done as you are able.

Know What You Can Control

Part of operating from strength is knowing what you can and cannot control. One of the most widespread complaints among people with chronic pain is loss of control. It starts with the inability to control what's happening in your body, which can escalate into being unable to control what's happening in your world. Pain is as unpredictable as your energy level, but you can still make choices and mobilize.

I want to steer you away from thinking about the losses or limitations facing you right now and toward the comforting territory of the things you still can do. Those are the things you can control. You're still in your family and in your world, so contribute to them as best you can. You still have interests and friends. Enjoy them.

The Benefits of Optimism

The greatest gift you will ever have is your life, and the second greatest gift—which you give yourself—is courage to live it to the fullest. Time goes by quickly; you cannot take it for granted.

Only you can create the true portrait of your life, with color, texture, feeling, spontaneity, and . . . your own fork! The simple truth is that *you* control what you think, what you say, how you feel, and how you behave. This takes courage, but it's the only way to be true to yourself and not let pain or other destructive forces steer you off your course. Since life is short, live it with optimism and joy.

CHAPTER 6

Drugs and Surgical Procedures

How Medication and Surgery Can Solve the Pain Puzzle

In my years as a medical practitioner, I've seen amazing traditional and complementary techniques that chip away at pain. Yet, with all the scientific breakthroughs in pain management, I've found that second only to going in for surgery, nothing worries people more than going on drug therapy! It's not because they don't want relief. It's because too many people hold on to fears or myths about drugs, so they may pass up a chance for real comfort.

To handle physical pain effectively, sometimes you need to take the right drug at the right dose, as monitored by your doctor. But because there are so many types of drugs for every level of pain, I'm going to offer you an overview of the different available drug therapies. At the same time, you can learn what these drugs can and cannot do for you—which will hopefully make it easier for you to discuss drug management with your doctor.

The Truth about Drug Addiction and Drug Dependency

It's impossible to talk about drugs without bringing up the number one myth: that by taking drugs, you become an addict. For people in chronic pain, many opiates are extremely effective; very few people become addicted. So before we get to the various drugs, let's talk about "addiction" and clear up what it really means. What is the fear all about?

Maybe you have ideas like these.

- "No drugs. I'll be in a daze all day."

- "I know what drugs do. A friend had to go to rehab for his addiction to painkillers. I'll stick to Tylenol."

- "I have an addictive personality. I took me 25 years to quit smoking and drinking. I'm not starting on any drug now!"

- "One drug leads to another. I won't be turned into an addict."

- "I'll take one pill a day at the lowest dose for 1 week. Then I'm off drugs for good."

In fact, these comments were all made by one patient over 2 months' time. Diana eventually changed some of these negative attitudes, but because of them, she endured unnecessary pain and worry. In every way, she expressed the many misconceptions about drugs that many people share—a fear of a knee-buckling addiction to a drug that might dull the pain but might also eventually control mind and body.

This was her story: By the time she turned 45, Diana's smoking habit led to lung disease. When I first treated her, she'd just been diagnosed with metastatic lung cancer. She complained of mild pains in her chest and around her liver, which was also affected. First I wanted to prescribe a weak opiate, like oxycodone plus acetaminophen (Percocet), which Diana was reluctant to take. She wanted relief, but her diagnosis stunned her. This is when she wanted to "stick to Tylenol." My sense was that Diana was in a state of denial and was still hoping she had a good chance to recover. Her choice of pain reliever reflected this state of mind: She held on to an over-the-counter preparation. Finally, the pain was beyond what Tylenol could control, and she agreed to take Vicodin.

When her pain got worse due to a mass pressing on nerves in her chest, Diana more readily upped her Vicodin dosage from four to six tablets a day. She began worrying about "addiction"; a friend's history of being addicted to painkillers led to concern that the same thing could happen to her. I assured her that this would not happen. Finally, her pain became exhausting and difficult for her to manage, and I recommended putting her on a long-acting drug. These types of drugs need to be taken only once or twice a day rather than four or more times a day.

So, knowing she would need such a drug, I suggested something very effective and inexpensive to treat the pain in her chest: low-dose methadone. Diana panicked. She said, "Are you kidding? It's for heroin addicts! I won't take it or I'll be floating around like a druggie."

Diana's story brings up a number of medications you've probably heard about: Percocet, Tylenol, Vicodin, methadone. Each one has a specific purpose, and each one can be either abused or used to best advantage, and to your benefit. But are they addictive?

When using opiates, there are three terms you need to be aware of: tolerance, physical dependence, and psychological dependence—now the preferred term for "addiction."

Tolerance is the escalating need for larger doses of medicine to maintain the desired effect. For example: Your doctor prescribed a medication that initially worked to relieve your pain for 8 hours, but now it works for only 6. You feel you need more medication.

The reality is that, clinically, tolerance to a drug doesn't exist if your condition or disease remains stable. You don't need more medicine unless your condition worsens. So if you have back pain due to arthritis, and the arthritis remains stable, whatever dose of opiates you're on will remain the same. If your arthritis gets worse, you need more medicine. Thus, tolerance doesn't occur unless there's a progression of the disease. It's not about the medication.

Physical dependence is an altered physical state produced by repeatedly taking a drug, which then necessitates taking it to prevent the appearance of withdrawal symptoms. The withdrawal symptoms vary by drug. Very simply, this is what I call the "coffee shop" phenomenon. For example, a woman drinks eight cups of coffee a day and then decides her caffeine intake is too great. She may not only cut back but cut coffee out completely. If she suddenly goes without the coffee her body is used to, she's going to endure a physical withdrawal from not having it. She'll get headaches, feel restless or anxious, have insomnia, or even feel depressed—all as part of the withdrawal from her physical dependence on coffee.

If you take steroids—drugs like Prednisone—you shouldn't stop them suddenly but instead ease off before stopping completely. If you're on antidepressants or an antihypertensive drug for high blood pressure, my advice is the same: You want to get off them slowly. If you taper off your medications slowly, you don't experience withdrawal, and it's not a problem. If you're on opiates for a long time, you *will* get a physical dependence, so again, you will need to wean yourself off them slowly.

Psychological dependence, or "addiction," is described as compulsive drug-seeking behavior with an overpowering involvement in procuring and using drugs. Experienced doctors very rarely confuse patients with pain asking for drug relief with people who have a history of chemical addiction and are seeking drugs for some sort of high.

Addiction, to be a bit more graphic, is like what's happening internally to the guy on the street stealing a TV set to buy narcotics. Think of crack addicts, who are chemically and psychologically in thrall to the drug. That's not like most people in pain, who, instead, are taking a medicine to which it is almost impossible to become addicted.

Which brings me back to Diana's faulty thinking that "one drug leads to another. I won't be turned into an addict." This is important to know: If you're in pain, the truth is that psychological dependence on any opiate treatment is very rare. Thus, true addiction is unlikely to happen to you, unless, as in some cases, you have a history of chemical dependence prior to taking a medication for real pain issues.

We all know people who have addictions and who use addictive substances for reasons other than to relieve physical pain. Nicotine and alcohol, or smoking and drinking, for example, provide psychological comfort. Diana's remark that she had "an addictive personality"—

specifically, that it took her 25 years to quit smoking and drinking—was very revealing. She was saying that if she could get addicted to cigarettes and bourbon, what could prevent her from becoming addicted to painkilling drugs?

Nicotine is considered to be physically addictive, and after about 72 hours of abstaining from it, it is completely eliminated from your system. After that, the urge for a cigarette is about ritual, comfort, pleasure, the heat of the stuff filling your lungs. There is a strong psychological dependence that occurs along with the physical one—despite the harm that your habit can do. If you're smoking, you know you're increasing your chances of lung or mouth or some other cancer related to tobacco use, and you continue to use it even though you know it is doing you harm. Recently, there were reports of people who abused dextromethorphan, an ingredient in over-the-counter cough syrups. Some of the people who dosed themselves with it for a high suffered serious consequences.

If you're using pain-abating opiates and you don't have real pain, you're addicted. But you're *not* addicted if you have pain. Instead, you're physically dependent, but only while on the drug.

People with a history of abusing drugs can still be treated with opiates for physical pain. However, these people need to be under strict medical supervision and usually need to sign a written contract with their physician. In fact, some pain centers will not write prescriptions without a contract. This contract is individualized and has at least the following terms of agreement: You agree that the doctor treating you with this drug is the *only* doctor prescribing this medication. You agree to get the medication from *only* one pharmacy. If you run out of the medication early, you agree not to get any refills without contacting the doctor first. There are even some pain centers that do random urine tests on patients taking prescribed drugs. If you violate the contract, the physician will usually discharge you from the clinic.

Some doctors ask every patient to sign a contract for certain opiates—whether or not they were or are drug addicts and no matter what their age or who they are. Contracts may be a bit controversial in the field of pain management, but many doctors find them necessary because there are so many people who are concerned about drugs.

Overall, exaggerated and unfounded fears of addiction shouldn't prevent you from taking an opiate your doctor recommends for chronic or severe pain. There have been many studies to prove that the benefits of taking opiates outweigh the potential for addiction.

Ultimately, Diana understood that life was still precious to her and that she wanted to get the most out of the time she had. She began methadone treatment and was surprised at how good she felt on it and how highly functioning she was. It was a smart decision.

Treating Pain with Over-the-Counter Preparations

We've all used drugstore products for pain relief, chief among them aspirin, acetaminophen (Tylenol), ibuprofen (Advil, Motrin), naproxen (Naprosyn, Aleve), and other similar medicines. Although many people think they're interchangeable, they're not. And even though you don't need a prescription for these pills, you need to treat them with respect. There are different maximum dosages for each, and each has either similar or different side effects you should be aware of.

When using over-the-counter (OTC) drugs, do not overlook the side effects just because these drugs are so easy to purchase. Have respect for all drugs, no matter how humble they seem to be; no drug should be taken lightly. If you have any questions, it is always best to check with your doctor.

Practitioners of pain management classify mild pain as Level 1 pain. You ache, and you're conscious of some discomfort, but you can function. You think, "I'll be fine" and don't bother calling your doctor. Instead, you self-treat with any one of many medications, usually beginning with aspirin.

Aspirin and Nonsteroidal Anti-Inflammatory Drugs

Aspirin is similar to a class of drugs called nonsteroidal anti-inflammatory drugs, or NSAIDs. It is sold under brand names such as Bayer, Excedrin, and Bufferin—as well as "house" brands sold in

QUESTIONS TO ASK YOUR DOCTOR ABOUT PAIN MEDICATION

- How much medicine should I take? How often?

- If my pain isn't relieved, can I take more medication? If the dose should be increased, by how much?

- Should I call you before increasing the dose?

- What if I forget to take my medication or take it too late?

- Should I take my medication with food?

- How much liquid should I drink with the medication?

- How long does it take the medicine to start working?

- Is it safe to drink alcoholic beverages, drive, or operate machinery after I have taken this medicine?

- What other medications can I take with the pain medicine?

- What side effects from the medication are possible, and how can I prevent them?

---

pharmacies or markets. Aspirin and NSAIDs work on somatic pain, especially achy, throbbing pain, such as the discomfort related to headaches, mild migraines, and arthritis. Sometimes one particular NSAID will work better for you than another. Talk to your doctor if you need greater relief. She may ask you to try other NSAIDs to figure out which one is best for your pain.

Types and common names: NSAIDs include ibuprofen, naproxen, piroxicam (Feldene), and oxaprozin (Daypro). One of the only NSAIDs that can be given by injection is ketorolac (Toradol), and this is usually given in the hospital after an operation.

Dosage: Always follow your doctor's directions regarding how

A CAVEAT FOR THREE NSAIDS

Most of the nonsteroidal anti-inflammatory drugs have what is called COX-1 and COX-2 activity. In recent years, three medications were developed that have COX-2 activity only: celecoxib (Celebrex), rofecoxib (Vioxx), and meloxicam (Mobic). These NSAIDs may produce less chance of gastrointestinal bleeding, but they have their downside. Recently, Vioxx was taken off the market because of the possibility of an increased risk of cardiac (heart) toxicity. It is possible that the same toxicity may ultimately be found with Celebrex and Mobic. Because of this potential side effect, these medications are no longer recommended for routine use.

many tablets to take during the day. For your own safety, carefully read the label on the bottle and do not exceed the daily dose that's recommended there. Overdosing on aspirin or nonsteroidal anti-inflammatory medications can lead to kidney failure and ulcers along with bleeding in the gastrointestinal tract.

Acetaminophen

Acetaminophen is well known by the brand name Tylenol. Acetaminophen is not in the same class as aspirin or NSAIDs. This popular pain reliever does help to reduce mild body pain, but it doesn't have very good anti-inflammatory properties, so it's not entirely clear to researchers how it works.

Acetaminophen is especially useful for treating pain when it is combined with certain opiates, such as oxycodone and hydrocodone. Acetaminophen is also often used as a pain reliever by pregnant women, but it's important for pregnant women to consult with their doctors before using any OTC medication.

Dosage: In many ways, acetaminophen is more dangerous than aspirin. People often think they can take more of it than is directed by the manufacturer because it is sold over the counter. It is a foolish presumption to think, "This stuff won't hurt me." If you overdose on acetaminophen, you can develop liver failure, which can lead to death. In general, it is not recommended to take more than 4 grams of acetaminophen per day, and no more than 3 grams for the elderly. Be sure to use it as directed on the medication's packaging. Unfortunately, there are no early warning symptoms of having taken too much, and overdosing can lead to coma.

When Over-the-Counter Medications Don't Work for You

I want to emphasize that physical pain can be handled effectively with the right drug at the right dose, but you *have* to take it as directed. If you've taken OTC drugs for 7 to 10 days, but they're not making you feel better, and your pain is becoming more chronic, you need to see an expert to figure out what's going on.

Chronic pain is not a treat-it-yourself project. Seeing a doctor gives you more accurate information and options. You'll know more about why you're having pain and what to do immediately to alleviate it—which may very well include prescription drugs.

Just as every person is different, every person's treatment regimen will be different. Your doctors will try to match the potency of the drug with the intensity of your pain. We want to make you feel better, but sometimes it takes trial and error—going from one drug to another—to see what makes the difference for you.

The Opiates

I once saw an amazing interview with Dennis Potter, the British writer who's mostly known for his quirky dramas, like *Pennies from Heaven*. Potter was suffering from a life-threatening disorder as well as from crippling arthritis that knotted his hands into fists and caused him great pain. Yet, with everything that ailed him, he was determined to be productive to the end—only a few months' time. Most of all, he wanted to finish a certain project, and he picked out the letters on a keyboard one at a time for a certain number of hours a day. To get through, Potter sought the help of his doctor.

With great feeling in his voice, Potter said that his doctor should be "celebrated" for "gently leading him to a balance between pain control and mental control" and to a space where he could work. One drug that helped was liquid morphine. I noticed with interest how clearheaded and upbeat Potter was and how he was equally articulate before and after taking the drug.

While Dennis Potter's condition was extreme, I know there are many of you out there who have days when you feel just as incapacitated by chronic pain. And while you're not at the end, you may be at the end of your rope. Drug therapy could be the answer for your chronic pain. Thus the next type of drugs for pain: the opiates. Here's an overview for you.

What Are Opiates?

Let me start by clarifying what is meant by opiates, which were formerly known as opioids or narcotics. An opiate is a drug that works on special receptors in the brain and spinal cord to relieve pain. These drugs work similarly to what we already produce in our brains, a group of hormones called endorphins.

Opiates are different from other medications. For example, one crucial difference between opiates and aspirin—or NSAIDs—is that aspirin and many NSAIDs have a ceiling for effectiveness. Because of that ceiling, higher doses of NSAIDs won't give you more pain relief, while higher doses of them *will* cause unwanted side effects. With opiates, you can, under a doctor's care, use as high a dosage as you need to control pain.

There is a wide range of "weak" and "strong" opiates and "short-acting" and "long-acting" opiates available in a number of different formulations. They can be taken in any number of ways: as tablets, in injectable and controlled-release forms, and in transdermal forms (drug-embedded patches applied to your skin).

The Weak Opiates

An opiate is considered to be weak if it is less potent than morphine, or if it works better when it's paired with another product, or "tagalong," like Tylenol or an NSAID. These weak opiates are still very effective for pain relief. They are short-acting formulations, which last from 3 to 4 hours per dose. This makes them particularly useful for breakthrough pain.

When I first see a patient with chronic pain, I recommend an opiate if I see that nothing else is helping. Often, people don't know that they need a stronger medication or how much to take. I recently treated a patient in her forties who came to see me about severe back pain. Georgia had tried physical therapy, acupuncture, chiropractic manipulation, massage, transcutaneous electrical nerve stimulator (TENS) treatment—the gamut of complementary protocols—and nothing worked for her. Her primary doctor prescribed tramadol, which she took faithfully, but it did not help the pain.

Because her pain got so bad, I wanted Georgia to switch medications and try the short-acting drug Percocet, which is acetaminophen and oxycodone. I suggested she take up to eight pills a day, every 4 to 6 hours, for 2 days. Then I started her on long-acting oxycodone (OxyContin). This regimen gave her long-term relief, and she was able to return to work as an accountant.

Types and common names: A few of the weak opiates are codeine, hydrocodone (Lortabs, Vicodin), oxycodone (Percocet, Percodan). Tramadol, often prescribed as a pain reliever, is not FDA approved as an opiate, though it could be considered a weak opiate since it works on opiate receptors in the brain.

Dosage: I would prescribe weak opiates for patients who are having less severe pain from ailments like arthritis and can be properly dosed with these drugs. Remember: With these opiates, more is *not* better. Weak opiates usually come in fixed oral doses with a nonopioid tagalong at a maximum safe dose.

The Strong Opiates

There are a number of strong opiates that are very helpful, if not life changing, for some pain patients.

Types and common names: Strong opiates include methadone, morphine, hydromorphone (Dilaudid), oxycodone, and fentanyl. There are two I would steer clear of: propoxyphene (Darvon,

Darvocet) and meperidine (Demerol). Research has shown that the metabolite of these two drugs can build up and lead to seizures and neurological complications. There have been literally hundreds of papers and reports about these complications.

Let's talk about methadone. This drug is best known as the substitute that is used to wean heroin addicts off the drug. It's an interesting medication that deserves more respect than it gets, mainly because it's a very good painkiller, and it's much cheaper than others.

One benefit is that methadone helps neuropathic, or nerve, pain.

While I see methadone coming more into favor, there are still many unfounded fears about it. One of my patients with rheumatoid arthritis was reluctant to start on methadone. Alan was in his midforties, had been married for 10 years, and had five children under the age of 8. He had been downsized out of his managerial job and had started a home business that hadn't quite taken off. He also watched the two youngest children, who were in school half a day. Then, because the children were so young, his wife cut down her hours as a bookkeeper to help take care of them.

I tried talking Alan into taking methadone because I knew it would help his pain, and it was actually the better drug for him. Also, because money was tight for Alan's family, I wanted to help him with his drug bills. His current prescriptions cost between $200 and $400 a month, while the cost of the same doses of methadone would be $15. This was a significant saving, but he refused, saying, "I'm not an addict. I won't take it and have people think it's my problem!" This attitude does Alan's well-being no good service.

Dosage: All strong opiates can ease your pain. What this means is that besides methadone, other good choices that may work for you as well are morphine, hydromorphone, oxycodone, and fentanyl. There is incomplete cross-tolerance between them, meaning that one may give you fewer side effects than another or may work better for your body. You will need to work with your doctor to try the different drugs until you find the one that's right for you.

The Adjuvants

The last drugs you need to be aware of for pain management are the adjuvants. These are medications that work with opiates to either increase their effectiveness, relieve their companion drugs' side effects, or treat nerve pain. Why take an adjuvant? Opiates usually take the edge off pain, but adjuvants are the helpers that will settle down the nerve, particularly in neuropathic pain, such as from shingles or diabetic neuropathy.

Anticonvulsants are the first line of adjuvants and are antiseizure medications. If you think about pain as a seizure of the nerve, in a sense, it's a nerve firing inappropriately. Gabapentin, carbamazepine, and valproic acid are just a few examples of adjuvants for this problem. There are always new anticonvulsants being tested, but these are currently the more common ones.

Tricyclic antidepressants are other first-line drugs for neuropathic pain. These drugs work by increasing serotonin in the brain. Two such drugs are amitriptyline (Elavil) and desipramine (Norpramin).

Every time you add a medication, you should expect some side effects. Medicate wisely.

Look at the list in "Common Drug Therapies for Pain" on page 152. It should help you sort out just some of the available drugs and the kind of pain they are usually prescribed for.

Managing the Possible Side Effects of Drugs

I understand how you feel when your doctor prescribes a drug for pain relief. On the one hand, you're probably eager to start the drug to feel better. On the other, you may be concerned about the drug itself. When I prescribe pain medicine, I often hear comments like:

- "What if I take this drug and fall asleep at the wheel?"

- "What if I can't keep food down?"

COMMON DRUG THERAPIES FOR PAIN

Mild to Moderate Pain

NSAIDs

Aspirin

Acetaminophen

Moderate to Severe Pain

Short-Acting Preparations

Codeine plus acetaminophen (Tylenol and codeine)

Hydrocodone plus acetaminophen or aspirin (Vicodin, Lortabs, Zydone, others)

Oxycodone plus acetaminophen or aspirin (Percocet, Percodan, Tylox, others)

Oxycodone, immediate release (Oxy IR, Roxicodone)

Morphine, immediate release

Hydromorphone (Dilaudid)

Oral transmucosal fentanyl citrate (Actiq)

Oxymorphone (in clinical development)

Long-Acting Preparations

Oxycodone, controlled release (OxyContin)

Morphine, controlled release (MS Contin, Kadian)

Methadone (Dolophine, others)

Fentanyl (Duragesic patches)

Oxymorphone (in clinical development)

- "What if the side effects make dealing with the pain even harder?"

If some uncomfortable side effects do not ease up over a certain amount of time, see your doctor. He will help you decide if it's best to manage the side effects of that drug or change prescriptions. Having certain side effects from one drug—like nausea—doesn't mean you'll get the same side effects from another drug. This is what we call incomplete cross-tolerance, meaning that even though a group of opiates are working on the same nervous system receptors, they don't necessarily affect everyone the same way. You may become nauseated or sedated from codeine but have no side effects from another opiate like hydrocodone or oxycodone. However, someone else may have completely different reactions.

Many people get side effects of sedation when they start on opiates. Those of us in pain management look at these side effects as typical and likely to go away or decrease in a week or so. In fact, I consider the feeling patients describe as being "logy" or "exhausted" or "doped" as exactly what it is: sleep deprivation catching up with them. You may be sleep deprived because severe pain has been keeping you awake or disturbing your sleep. Take an opiate, and you don't have pain any more. You suddenly fall asleep the second your head touches the pillow, and you might even sleep for 2 days straight! You wake rested, but while you're sleeping, the folks around you may go nuts with worry and keep checking on you to make sure you're breathing.

It's not uncommon for a family member to call me, worried that the opiate is too strong. Let me assure you and those who love you that sleeping for longer stretches will go away in time and that this is not a problem. If the sleepiness doesn't lessen, there are medications that can help. Your sleeping longer may make your family wonder if you'll be totally in a haze and unable to function. This is a myth. Think of Dennis Potter in his last days, productive on painkilling drugs. This is why a positive "keep your fork" attitude is so important. Drugs are part of the dynamic pain management mix. The primary goal of opiate therapy for patients in chronic pain is to make them more functional, not to slow them down.

Nausea and vomiting sometimes occur, but there are medications to treat these symptoms. If you take opiates with food and not on an empty stomach, you reduce the chances of stomach upsets. If the nausea doesn't go away, you can change to another opiate that may not cause this side effect for you. Unfortunately, one side effect that remains constant is constipation. Since I know patients are very likely to get it, I usually put them on a regimen that prevents and treats constipation by moving the bowels along—something like senna or some form of fiber product and a stool softener. Getting constipated is not a reason to decline opiates, especially since prevention and treatment are so easy and accessible.

Other than sleepiness, nausea, vomiting, and constipation, sometimes people experience itchiness or confusion. A very, very rare side effect is respiratory depression, which means you can't breathe properly. This won't happen if your medication is given in the correct dosages. If you experience breathing problems, get medical assistance immediately.

Interventional Pain Treatments: Anesthetic Procedures and Neurosurgical Techniques

When medication over the long run is not effective for pain relief, the answer for you may be an interventional or invasive procedure. This not only means surgery but can also include an anesthetic procedure or technique. Research in this field is ongoing, and every month or so, we read about a hopeful treatment that's still in experimental stages. For now, let me tell you about a few possibilities that may be tried for some of the most common pain syndromes.

Anesthetic and neurosurgical procedures are usually performed by anesthesiologists, neurologists, or neurosurgeons and are done when other, more conservative management of a pain problem does not work. The procedures are always invasive and are always done under careful monitoring by medical specialists. Such procedures can sometimes be done on an outpatient basis, while on other occasions you will need to be in the hospital for a few days.

Is a neurosurgical or anesthetic interventional approach right for you? Of course, speak to your primary care doctor or pain doctor about your options for pain relief in these categories. Your doctor will know when such intervention is called for and which choice might be best for you. Listed below are only some of the possible procedures used.

Epidural steroids. This treatment often helps people who have herniated disks that cause immobilizing pain. For this procedure, your doctor injects a steroid into the target epidural space in your back. This procedure doesn't require a hospital check-in overnight but is done in a hospital surgical center. For some people, these treatments can relieve the pain for months. However, you may need a series of three injections to get the full benefit.

Cryosurgery. For this procedure, the doctor freezes the nerve. Cryosurgery can be especially helpful for people who have developed neuromas, which are growths on nerve cell sheaths that cause nerves to become entangled and fire oddly. These growths often develop where people have scars from previous surgeries.

Dorsal column stimulator. This is an option for some people who have chronic back pain that radiates down their legs. People who try this intervention usually do so because they can't find relief with drug therapy. A dorsal column stimulator is an implant that works on the spinal level to help control pain by sending electrical impulses up the spinal cord.

Intrathecal pump. Doctors may suggest an intrathecal pump if a dorsal column stimulator fails. This is a little battery-operated device about the size of a pacemaker. A catheter is inserted into the spine, and the pump itself is implanted in the subcutaneous fat (below the skin) in your abdomen. Medications such as opiates and local anesthetics (numbing medicines like bupivacaine) are infused via this pump to control pain.

I recently met a Connecticut osteopath with a long history of bone pain who came to a lecture I gave on pain management. Dave was in his midfifties and told me that he finally had a time when he felt healthy and normal, only because he'd had an intrathecal pump put in.

Since he was 20 years old, Dave had come to have arthritis in his back and problems with his legs and back from a degenerative disk disease called spinal stenosis. With this disorder, there's a narrowing of the spinal canal along with an increase of bony tissue—Mother Nature's defense, much like developing a callus on your skin because you're irritating it. Dave learned to adapt and function around the pain. In fact, he was married 10 years before his wife knew how much pain he was in. "I played an ego game that wound up hurting me more," he told me.

For a long time, Dave wouldn't take any medication stronger than aspirin, worrying that they would make him logy when he treated his patients. He'd also read an article about some doctors getting addicted to drugs, and he was determined he wouldn't be one of them. With all his pain, he still played tennis, taking the pain as a "burden" and only stopping physical activities when it was too excruciating to continue.

As Dave got older, his spinal stenosis got worse, as did his degenerative arthritis. He reached a stage where he couldn't walk because of the arthritis, and he had two hip replacements, which, he said, "helped his hip pain wonderfully" but did not help his pain from spinal stenosis. He was placed on strong opiates and adjuvant medications, which didn't help. At that point, the decision was made to place an intrathecal pump.

Scientific advancements often come along just in time. I asked him about his decision to have the pump implanted. He said, "If you asked me when I had the least amount of pain, it would be in the last 2 years, thanks to this implant." With pain relief, Dave not only feels better, he can function better. For him, the intrathecal pump is a miracle. Pain once affected every part of his life, and now he is thankful for being alive and nearly pain free.

A Final Reminder about Taking Medication

Your best bet is to always fully understand any treatment that involves drugs or interventional treatment before you agree to it. Drugs have potencies, dosages, and side effects to consider.

Interventional treatments are usually invasive to some degree and require recovery time.

Most of all, with drug therapy for pain, remember this: If one drug doesn't work for reducing your pain, talk to your doctor about trying another. This is what doctors call doing "sequential trials," and it is perfectly normal. Don't give up, thinking that all drugs are the same. Find what's best for you to stay pain free.

CHAPTER 7

Complementary Medicine

How Nontraditional Therapies
Can Make a Difference in How You Feel

Nontraditional therapies offer a number of real possibilities for alleviating the many problems associated with pain. In my crusade to help people relieve their pain, my "army" of forces for pain relief includes hands-on systems like Reiki, stress management techniques, music and art therapies, acupuncture, hypnosis, and biofeedback. Uppermost among the benefits of these therapies may be temporary relief from chronic pain.

Although I've been schooled in traditional medicine, I'm enough of a believer in many complementary modalities to suggest you try them. I define complementary medicine as treatments and therapies that are used in addition to drugs and other traditional medical procedures. Many of them, such as Reiki and acupuncture, have certainly helped me. Medically unorthodox, or nontraditional, therapies appeal to people who either do not like taking prescription drugs but need to, or those who like supplementing medication and physical therapy with other pain-control techniques.

However, I do not recommend you use these (and other) nontraditional treatments and therapies as *alternative* medical care. By this I mean treatments or therapies that you embrace *instead of* and *to the exclusion of* traditional medical care. So, if you had fibromyalgia, for example, I could not suggest that you get treatment from only a massage therapist, a nutritionist, or any other such practitioner. If so, you would be undergoing alternative medical care. If you were being treated by an accredited physician as your primary doctor who also recommended massage therapy, nutritional counseling, or another such practice, you would be in a complementary medical program.

Are complementary therapies right for you? Do they interest you? Baffle you? Be assured that many therapies are worth a try. Surveys show that many people are willing to try complementary techniques and that they are no longer an unusual option. One in four patients uses some form of alternative therapy instead of traditional medicine, and, unfortunately, the majority of those patients don't inform their primary doctors. For example, I know of people who stop taking their prescription medication without telling their doctors. Meanwhile, they try out an alternative treatment, such as herbal brews or coffee enemas, allegedly meant to target, manage, or cure their disorder. Not smart.

However, the number of visits by patients who use either complementary or alternative therapies now exceeds those of patients going to primary care doctors alone. Now, more people than ever are using a combination of traditional medicine and complementary techniques (as I do). The number of people who see only a traditional primary care doctor is decreasing. Ten years ago, they were the majority—more people then followed "doctor's orders" only and shrugged off nontraditional approaches.

In the last 25 years or so, there has been a greater interest in—and acceptance of—investigating pain control through complementary modalities. If you are dealing with chronic pain, such modalities can help you feel more in charge of your body and your life. A good pain-control program will address the psychological as well as physiological realities of your pain problems and is worth checking into through your doctor.

There is no doubt that complementary techniques can reduce or relieve pain in some measure. My experience is that people use less medication when they start using some of the techniques I'll talk about shortly. No matter how small the effect, it's worth a try!

The Growing Popularity of Complementary Therapies

Many of what are now considered accepted alternative therapies were once the only source of practical medical treatments. They co-exist now with supersophisticated pharmaceutical and surgical techniques for treating pain. In a very real way, complementary therapies describe medical progress.

About 100 years ago, before there were medicine chest staples like aspirin or ibuprofen or prescription painkilling drugs, it was not unusual to hear of people taking laudanum, a tincture of opium, to relieve their pain. Others tried nonmedical treatments like hot sweat baths with massage, hoping to perspire away the pain and relieve muscle cramping. A rubdown or "salt glow" following the bath was concentrated on a sore area to stimulate blood flow. "Galvanism," a less fearsome cousin of shock treatment, applied electrical current to the area to reduce pain. Along with the staple of family recipes for healing that were handed down from generation to generation, liniments, decoctions, poultices, and brews were available from doctors, mail-order catalogs, pharmacies, and quacks selling "miracles" in a jar.

Then there's now.

Modern pharmacology can manufacture drugs using synthetics, plants, minerals, and chemistry, but until this development was technically possible, people relied on plants. In fact, more than 100 conventional drugs are manufactured from them. Since the late 1960s, there's been a growing interest in herbs, and what's old is new again. You can get essential oils extracted from plants or vaporized for aromatherapy. There are topical products (applied to the skin) that can reduce inflammation or, as with capsicum oleoresin, produce anesthesia. Herbs are serious stuff, and the fact that they are "natural" doesn't mean they are free of adverse side effects when you ingest them. If you have any other condition, like high blood pressure or diabetes, be sure you know how the herb may affect you before taking it.

Galvanism has grown up, too, into space-age, electrically based devices and applied techniques that continue to change lives. The pacemaker, implanted in heart patients, is one. Pain patients, especially those with arthritis and back pain, can now opt for TENS (transcutaneous electrical nerve stimulation), which utilizes an electrical stress- and pain-control unit. TENS units are put on a patient's back or another spot on the body for the purpose of pain relief. It works by confusing the nervous system through its electrical activity. And while it may sound impossible, major medical research centers are studying the positive effects of magnetism. Some of these therapies require the ministrations of experts on an individual basis. Others, like music, art therapy, and yoga, can be incorporated into your daily life and done either with a practitioner or on your own.

Why Choose Complementary Therapies?

Patients always ask me if such therapies are right for them. Before answering, I have to know more about how they feel and think about some of the nontraditional techniques I just described. What always proves true is that you will definitely maximize the benefits from complementary therapies if:

• You are attracted to them.

• You tend to believe in them or are willing to suspend your doubts or apprehensions about these techniques working for you.

• You prefer to be actively engaged in doing what you can outside of and alongside mainstream medical approaches.

A good measure of satisfaction comes from having some success with these complementary techniques, since many of them depend on your commitment to them in time, energy, and a sense of purpose. Unlike conventional medical therapies, they can be something of a challenge in this regard, but they are nonetheless fascinating.

When you learn how complementary therapies can help heal pain, you will understand more about who you are while also having the adventure of mastering a new discipline such as meditation and yoga.

Because there is so much written about them, let me describe just a few of the therapies I tend to use most or recommend in my practice. They fall into the main categories determined by the National Center for Complementary and Alternative Medicine. The chart below shows what you'll find in the first four categories, most of which I have used myself or recommended for my patients.

There are a number of options in each category for you to choose from. Let's examine them, starting with the 5,000-year-old practice of acupuncture.

COMPLEMENTARY PAIN THERAPIES

Alternative Medical Systems	Mind-Body Interventions	Manipulative and Body-Based Therapies	Energy Therapies
Acupuncture	Guided imagery	Yoga	Reiki
—	Hypnosis	Tai chi	Therapeutic touch
—	Biofeedback	Qigong	Magnet therapy
—	Meditation	Massage	—
—	Spiritual guidance and prayer	Osteopathic manipulation	—
—	Music, art, and dance therapies	Chiropractic	—

Acupuncture

With its basis in Taoist philosophy, acupuncture first struck Western observers as little more than Chinese folklore or "barefoot medicine." Most American doctors were dubious about the scientific credibility of this ancient medical system, equating it with superstitious kitchen cures like chicken soup for colds or pickle juice for removing warts.

However, over 3 decades ago, acupuncture was introduced in a dramatic way to America: An American journalist, stricken with appendicitis upon his arrival in Peking, agreed to postoperative acupuncture to relieve abdominal pain. An hour after conventional surgery, and with acupuncture treatments, he felt free of abdominal pressure. Subsequently, teams of American doctors toured Chinese medical centers to observe the alleged range of acupuncture's capabilities, beyond that of inducing anesthesia. What they found, among other things, was that acupuncture treatments could raise the level of bacteria-fighting white blood cells, thereby arming the body to more efficiently fight disease.

How does acupuncture work? In China, this needle-based therapy developed in conjunction with the accompanying practice of moxibustion, or the burning of the herb mugwort, at or near the appropriate points on the patient's body. According to Chinese theory, disease is an imbalance of yin (female) and yang (male) forces disrupting an orderly flow of qi (pronounced "chi"), or energy. Bodily organs, as well as behavior, temperature, and other functions, are assigned yin or yang attributes. Even the ingestion of food is based on this principle of opposites. There are yin foods (such as fruit) and yang foods (such as meat) as well as foods that are balanced (such as brown rice).

Acupuncturists take as truth the theory energy flows from organ to organ through channels, or meridians, beneath the skin. There are 12 such meridians running on either side of the body and 1 along the center, front and back. There are about 360 anatomic points spaced along these meridians that an acupuncturist must learn to pierce with needles, thereby correcting imbalances in the corresponding organs. Once the needles are in place, they may be twirled or not, depending on the complex law governing the relationship between the type of needling and the organs.

So, what happens next? No one can quite explain how it happens, but the needling may unblock a channel and release stagnated energy or—usually more important for pain sufferers—reduce the sensations of pain and cramping.

Should you try this ancient therapy as a complement to taking medication or doing physical therapy as suggested by your doctor? Or would you opt for acupuncture as your sole therapy? Acupuncture is a relatively benign therapy that may help in some cases for your pain management. However, part of a positive acupuncture treatment is going in willing to believe that it can help you. Some pain patients tell me that they get very little relief from acupuncture treatments, while others go eagerly for the next experience. Understand that you may get the benefit of some immediate decrease in pain, headaches, and nausea; however, it's more likely that you'll need a series of consecutive treatments before you feel better.

Patients always ask me if the "needling" hurts. In general, it's not painful, but some people find the insertion of the needles uncomfortable. This discomfort may have to do with where on your body the acupuncturist inserts the needles and in what state of health you are.

There is a lot of research on acupuncture that shows it helps. It is an accepted modality nowadays, and more and more insurance companies are paying for the treatments. Acupuncture is so accepted now that the FDA has removed acupuncture needles from its experimental device category, choosing instead to regulate them as mainstream medical devices. Although it has grown immensely in popularity as a pain-relieving treatment, acupuncture still has its mystique—but remember, it's not a cure. If acupuncture sounds right for you, be sure that the practitioner you go to is licensed, experienced, and recommended.

Guided Imagery and Hypnosis

With guided imagery, you are helped to picture yourself in your mind's eye feeling safe, happy, and pain free. The next step up from guided imagery is hypnosis. During hypnosis, you are led to a state of relaxation through calming and repetitive suggestions from a practitioner, causing you to reach a different level of consciousness.

Biofeedback

A biofeedback machine allows you to see how your heart and respiratory rates go down as you either listen to or tell yourself repetitive suggestions to relax. You see evidence of your efforts on the monitor as you concentrate on increasing your alpha brain wave levels, which indicate whether you're relaxing.

Who's right for biofeedback? A patient came to see me suffering with severe pain from prostate cancer. Lou told me that he wanted something to do to reduce his pain level. As I was asking him what he'd been considering, Lou opened his briefcase and pulled out charts of his PSA levels, which had gone up over the last few months. (PSA stands for prostate specific antigen, which is a blood marker that sometimes increases when men have prostate cancer.) He wanted to know, as his PSA went up, what part of his body would feel pain. I knew that Lou was a man who would not do well with hypnosis or any other free-form imagery technique. He clearly was comfortable with data, graphs, and charts; felt as if he could control his pain by monitoring it; and would actually enjoy seeing the biofeedback machines in operation. Biofeedback did, indeed, help Lou. Although he was a skeptic at first, he later looked forward to his sessions.

Meditation

I sometimes think of meditation as an exercise in focusing on inner peace. Inner peace is already there for you, but you need to access it. Meditation is one way.

Meditation was brought to the Western world from India by the Maharishi Mahesh Yogi in the late 1960s. This guru, or spiritual leader, taught a mind-control technique known as TM, or transcendental meditation. Unlike yoga and acupuncture, which are rooted in more religious systems and philosophies, meditation is considered a natural approach to reducing stress, inducing therapeutic healing, and expanding awareness.

TM's relaxation techniques help alter brain waves, control heart rate, stimulate circulation, and decrease muscle tension. Meditation is also known to reduce or eliminate anxiety attacks, gastrointestinal problems, and many other psychological and physical effects that come from high-stress living. In fact, researchers investigating TM's beneficial qualities found fewer sleep disturbances (which is especially helpful to many pain sufferers) and even improved learning ability and general mental health.

That's quite a menu of benefits! How does TM work to effect such a range of changes? To meditate, you sit with your eyes closed and your feet flat on the floor, preferably in a silent room, although many practitioners can meditate in public places, including planes, waiting rooms, and doctor's offices. To help bring about the paradoxical state of deep rest with increased wakefulness, you must shift your awareness inward and tune out the environment. This sensation has been likened to the near-suspension of complete consciousness before falling asleep. To aid in concentration, some people picture an imaginary spot on their foreheads and focus on that; others may disengage from the outside world by either silently or vocally repeating a word that has been especially selected for them by a TM instructor. This sound syllable, such as the widely used "om," is called a mantra.

TM is a good relaxation technique, best practiced twice a day for about 15 minutes each time. Even if you try this technique once a day, it may help you relax and relieve pain. To help you to get into the meditative mood, seek out tapes and CDs that guide you through the process or provide meditative-quality background music.

Arts Therapies

I feel confident in saying that expressing creativity is one of the most engaging, if not most powerful, acts we can do for ourselves.

Creativity produces wonderful results in the shape of paintings, crafts, songs, dances, journals, and music. Creativity is also healing, and it reaches levels that medication doesn't. Part of our spiritual dimension, it connects to who we are at the deepest level.

Many of my patients have discovered abilities and talents during music and art therapy sessions that they didn't know they had or didn't have time to work on—and at the same time, found a singular sense of pain relief in the creative act itself. You're not going for a brilliant end result but instead are seeking the pleasure of losing yourself in positive self-expression and moving away from your pain. You can also disconnect temporarily from your troubles while enjoying music and art. It's what happens when you go to a concert, for example, and find yourself so involved in the music that both time and troubles are suspended. That you leave feeling elevated and in high spirits is a bonus.

This is exactly what you want to tap into with arts therapies. Sheila Egan, who is a music therapist, understands how her specialty benefits pain patients. She started out singing with a small opera company and later became a voice teacher and a practitioner of Reiki. In her job, she's seen how music changes consciousness or reduces pain levels for patients with chronic illnesses. She explains why some patients may not be interested in music or art therapy: "For one thing, when a patient is in chronic pain, they get into a pain, loop and can't get out of it. They panic about being in pain, and it's all they can focus on, especially if they're bedridden, which many are where I work. What I do is find out what kind of music they like and work with it in all kinds of activities."

Egan once worked with a patient who had a devastating disease that, among other symptoms, caused large, painful lesions all over his body. When she met him, Charlie was only 18 years old and depressed, and he wouldn't get out of bed to get his blood circulating. She knew Charlie liked blues and 1970s rock and roll, so she decided to tempt him to sit up and play an electric drum machine. "It's set up with drum pads and not as noisy as regular drum sets, and you can put a headset on and listen to your playing," she said. "I brought the drum set to Charlie's room, and it got him up and out of bed. Most important, it distracts him from his pain. He can sit and play for hours."

Whether it's through music, art, drama, or writing, tap into your creative center. It will never let you down.

Yoga

One first associates this ancient Indian discipline with its most famous symbol, the lotus position, a sitting posture with legs folded in a pretzel shape. Yoga is far more than just a series of such very specific postures, though. It is also, like acupuncture, based on a philosophical system that encompasses cosmic ideologies, theories about life forces and one's control over them, and healing.

For one thing, yoga teaches its practitioners to concentrate on deep and rhythmic breathing, which is instrumental for inducing relaxation and an overall sense of well-being. If you are physically able to get into the postures without causing undue stress on your bones and muscles, yoga can help you. If you are unable to get into and sustain the postures, you may still benefit from following along and concentrating on yogic breathing techniques.

Yoga concentrates on taking in prana, or the vital force that is assimilated into the body through breath control. Prana is meant to quiet the mind by diminishing awareness of the external environment. Those who are very practiced at the breathing art, such as a yogi or any expert devotee of the discipline, can learn to drastically slow down their breathing rate as well as alter consciousness to the point of inducing a trance state. But for most of us, yoga breathing techniques offer a means to a pleasant sense of tranquility and pain relief.

Breathing technique is an essential part of doing yoga postures, or asanas. These asanas are designed to strengthen the back, tone the muscles, increase flexibility, stimulate nerves and glands, change the direction of blood flow, help in the elimination of waste products, and oxygenate the body through slow breathing. These exercises do not "go for the burn" like energetic aerobics, weight training, or pedaling a stationary bike. Instead, nearly all the postures are static, held for a period of time while breathing rhythmically.

Yoga is best learned at first with a teacher's guidance rather than through a book. It looks easy and sounds simple, but you will get more out of it with the help of an expert and with the permission of a doctor, especially if you have back, neck, or joint pain. Of course, an expert can give you smart and knowledgeable tips about body alignment and show you how to get in and out of the postures safely and properly. Yoga classes are frequently offered through adult education programs and at many YMCAs, local gyms, dance studios, and of course, yoga centers, where classes are conducted by people who have mastered the system. You can also find yoga instruction videos, but again, don't try any postures on your own without first consulting with your doctor.

Massage

Massage helps people in many ways, whether or not they have chronic pain issues. Massage is practically *de rigeur* for athletes after a game or a match, and for good reason: Massage is noninvasive and calming, it gets circulation going, and it relaxes taut or sore muscles. Some people worry about getting a vigorous massage, in which the masseur or masseuse kneads the muscles as part of the session. However, I've seen patients with myofascial pain or conditions in which muscles are taut or strained helped immensely by such a rubdown. A real laying on of hands, massage helps people calm down and relieves anxiety.

There are different styles of massage, such as deep-tissue or Swedish massage. Trigger-point release massage is done by rehab doctors, podiatrists, and anesthesiologists. It works by placing a needle into the muscle to help release it if massage alone doesn't work. Studies show it is effective in decreasing pain and its associated symptoms. The choice of which style of massage to try is yours to make after consulting your doctor.

Reiki

I'm a true believer in Reiki, a calming, gentle hands-on technique that I use for myself and recommend when it seems appropriate. Reiki is a fairly new complementary technique developed by a Japanese doctor who, while on a spiritual quest to understand hands-on healing and why it worked, put together the system called Reiki.

Reiki means "universal life force." The practice isn't massage but is based on spiritual energy. Reiki practitioners believe that they can draw energy from the universal life force around them and then let it flow through their hands and into the person who needs to be healed. This energy also releases blockages that can prevent you from healing. With Reiki, there's no risk of adding to your aches or pains, and it is safe for young and old. In this healing system, the practitioner is considered a channel through which energy is drawn into a patient.

The Reiki practitioner uses specific hand positions that correspond to the body's organs, to the body's emotional and dynamic properties, and to the location of seven chakras. These chakras are centers of concentrated energy that supposedly vibrate over specific areas. Reiki hand positions are meant to create balance in the chakras and energy fields.

For example, one of the chakras is the root chakra, which is a spot located at the base of the spine and connected to the adrenals, bladder, genitals, and spine and to the life force. Another is the solar plexus chakra, which connects to the pancreas, liver, and stomach and to the qualities of power, fear, and control.

By laying hands on various parts of the body, the practitioner can transmit energy to help restore the natural flow. The person in pain responds and relaxes. Landis Vance, the chaplain mentioned earlier, explains it best. "There's no manipulation of the body, so it's not like deep-tissue massage or chiropractic or any other more vigorous system. It's not a religious system, yet you can't help feeling an emotional release and a spiritual connection to what is happening."

A benefit of a Reiki treatment is understanding that you need to take responsibility for your healing through adopting a more positive mental and emotional attitude. Reiki practitioners follow a value system based on simple human dignity, as they would say, applied "just for today." This system's tenets include not worrying so that your mind is "easy," being at peace and not getting angry, earning an honest living and doing no harm to anyone, and showing gratitude to every living being and their ability to grow and understand others.

Is Reiki for you? If you have a lot of anxiety and spiritual distress, and nothing is quite relieving your pain, including counseling or hypnosis, Reiki may be a real option. I use Reiki a lot when it's clear that we have to get to another level of the patient's consciousness to be able to help.

Neal is a good example. I was treating Neal when he was 20 years old. He had had a bone marrow transplant for leukemia and suffered with a lot of pain in his legs. He was especially distressed because his younger brother was going off to college on a partial football scholarship. While he didn't begrudge his brother's good fortune, it made him aware that he might never get to a game to see his brother play or be able to run around a field, strong and healthy, again.

He was one sick young man whose anxiety seemed unrelieved. We treated Neal's pain with a variety of opiates and an anticonvulsant, but drugs weren't getting to the underlying issue. "I can't do relaxation stuff," he'd say, dismissing our efforts to encourage him to try complementary therapies. I suggested Reiki. It differs from some other techniques in that you're not really talking things out and increasing stress, and you're not actively doing anything except lying in bed while the practitioner manipulates the energy fields within and around you.

My recommendation turned out well. Neal's anxiety lessened after a number of treatments. Happily, he was eventually able to stop living in a state of fear about what would happen to him next and to allow himself the gift of peace of mind. He still comes in once a month for follow-up Reiki treatments to maintain the level of spiritual peace that he struggled to achieve.

Magnets

Don't ask me how they work, but I believe that magnets can make a difference in reducing pain. Some medical specialists call magnetism quackery, but I wouldn't give up on magnet therapy until the results of the studies are in.

Interest in magnets was aroused by the number of reports from people who said they had less or no pain after having an MRI (magnetic resonance imaging) scan. The MRI machine itself is, in effect, a large and powerful magnet.

As someone with disk problems, I'm inclined to try anything that helps me without altering my consciousness at work. Thus, I wear a belt loaded with little magnets and feel better some of the time. You don't have to wear such a belt, but you can buy little magnets at some chain drugstores, some health food stores, and stores that sell herbs, as well as from specialty Internet sites. You don't want to use refrigerator magnets or any magnet that's been painted or has (or had) anything made of plastic or synthetic glued onto it. Paint, glue, and synthetics tend to block the flow of energy.

Since the magnets are small, you'll need to create some sort of simple rigging to keep them in place. You can usually find the appropriate belts or rigging where you find the magnets, or again, check the specialty Internet sites for magnet therapies. Or you can make a fabric "tube," similar to the channel at the top of a curtain to slip the rod into.

A Final Word on Complementary Techniques

People are now so much more educated about complementary medicine than ever before and can make smart choices about their health care. I've seen so many patients respond to the techniques in this chapter that I want to put in a final word of encouragement for you to try one. Will complementary therapies alone relieve pain? Probably not. But because these techniques offer benefits like eliminating or reducing nausea, vomiting, anxiety, sleep disorders, and muscle pain and increasing a sense of well-being, it's a good idea to try a therapy today.

If any of these therapies interest you, *always* consult with your doctor before leaping into a modality and hoping for the best. You must be sure that the modality doesn't conflict with the treatments or medication you're taking. To find reputable practitioners, check with the hospital your doctor is connected with, since many hospitals now have complementary or integrative medical departments. If your doctor or the hospital near you cannot recommend or provide a specific practitioner, check out the Appendix under "Building a Team: Where to Find Medical Professionals." There you'll find a list of organizations you can contact for information on exactly what kind of credentials the practitioner of choice is required to have and how to find a practitioner in your area.

CHAPTER 8

Caregiving

What the People Who Care about You
Should Know

I am still learning how people make sense of pain. I may not have an explanation that would satisfy everyone, but I do know that what another person thinks and feels about pain may not necessarily make sense to you or me. There are so many factors that go into understanding and accepting pain that it's easy to see why we'd be confused or unsure of why others feel as they do. Nowhere are these personal discrepancies as pronounced as in an intimate setting where caregivers are nonprofessionals—such as relatives and friends. While they're there to help you through, they can feel unsure of themselves, or even helpless, in such a situation.

When I talk about caregiving, people automatically think of the routines that need to be followed, such as giving medication, trips to the doctor or some therapy session, or even how to set up a bedroom or living room so that the person in pain can get around more easily. But caregiving is a lot more than a series of medically based or mundane tasks that need to be performed and attended to. The most important aspect of caregiving is the relationship between the caregiver and the person being cared for. It is this relationship that can intensify caring between two people and even add a spiritual dimension to the caregiving ritual.

I've stressed spirituality and increasing intimacy with others throughout this book as part of your healing process, and caregiving can take it to a finer point. A caregiver is anyone who devotes time and effort to help you relieve your pain so you can function better. This can be a spouse, a parent, a good friend, a nurse, a therapist of any kind (physical or psychological), or a health-care assistant who is hired on a part- or full-time basis. At their best, caregivers are reliable, and they can use their intellectual approach to caretaking. At their most gifted, they bond with you, and their care gains depth and greater meaning.

As no doctor can understand the degree of your pain if you hold back information, the same is true for caregivers. Thus, the relationship between you and the person who wants to care for you begins with the fine art of communication. Let's look at how you can promote healing by improving your relationships with caregivers and how caregivers can feel more assured about helping you when you're in pain.

Relating to a Caregiver When You're in Pain

Communication can be hard enough in a very busy world when you're healthy, but it's much tougher when you're in pain. There are ways to narrow the communication gap—as long as everyone concerned is willing to open up just enough. Shutting down cannot help you and keeps the people who want to help you at a disadvantage. I have a few ideas for you to consider.

The Power of Talking It Out

I had a call from an associate who asked me to see a relative of his who worried him. Kate, who is in her early forties, seemed to have a good life, until she fell and hurt herself. She said she had simply gotten out of her car and started walking up her driveway at home when she lost her footing and fell, literally, on her face. There was some bruising, but no broken skin or bones. Kate had some nerve pain, and although she was having a difficult time dealing with it, she was still functioning as she did normally on a daily basis: as a wife, mother, and working professional. She had been married for 15 years to a successful businessman, her three children were healthy and doing well in school, and she worked as an accountant for a large firm.

Kate's husband was concerned about her and took her to the hospital for tests. No neurologist could find any reason for her fall, so she next consulted with a rheumatologist, who is specialized to diagnose lupus, arthritis, and fibromyalgia. Kate tested negative for all three disorders and was given painkillers for the nerve pain she felt, especially on one side of her face.

Then, 4 months later, she fell twice more—both times on her driveway, both times on the way to her front door. There was no ice or cracked cement on the driveway when she fell, and she explained the falls by saying her heel gave out under her, and the packages she was carrying pulled her down.

That's when my associate called, asking for my advice. Kate's pain had progressed from her face to her left arm, and she had started on methadone for pain relief. After the third fall, she'd lapsed into feeling total body pain, to the point where she could not get out of bed. I call this a total shutdown.

What was going on in Kate's life? Since I did not treat her from the beginning, I could not pinpoint the dramatic switch from "This is how my life goes" to "I don't want to live this life anymore because it's too painful!" Why had a woman who seemingly had a nice life changed from a highly functioning person into someone who suddenly had to stop in her tracks. I spoke to her once, and my immediate goal was to relieve her pain and restore some of her normal activities. I thought that therapy and acupuncture treatments could really help her, and she very quietly acquiesced. I made appointments for her with a psychotherapist and an acupuncture doctor, but she canceled both at the last minute, calling me to say she was too exhausted to get to either place. I asked her to come to see me in my office. She said she'd get back to me, but she hasn't so far.

While Kate had a number of caregivers who were totally behind her healing process, she was in rejection mode. As it turned out, she rejected her husband's efforts to figure out what was wrong with her, and she wouldn't tell him what doubts or fears she may have had about their marriage. Did she feel as if she'd failed as a wife, mother, or professional, or as a person? Did she want to leave her marriage but force herself to stay by causing herself injury? Did she want to give up her high-pressure job and stay at home to raise her children but feel guilty because they needed her income to maintain their lifestyle?

Kate wasn't talking, nor was she allowing anyone into her orbit who could break through her emotional agony, help heal her physical pain, and stop what could be more serious falls in the future. Furthermore, by canceling appointments that I'd made for her, she stayed stuck at a point that distressed and confused not only her but also those who wished to help her. To me, Kate had many psychosocial issues that she hadn't confronted, and they were literally tripping her up. She was in total pain, and she isolated herself from her caregivers—very unwise!

Communication is not just an exchange of information or one person answering the questions of another. It's not about assuming what others must feel because you "know" them or they "know" you. It's not speaking for someone else. It's not aggressively accusing someone in pain of slacking off in the hopes of propelling them out of their condition and into wellness.

The Elements of Communication

Ideally, real communication demonstrates an ability to speak truthfully about how you feel, to really listen, to show empathy and hear between the lines, and to make an effort to accept—if not understand—what the other person is saying. Sounds daunting! I know all of these elements may appear difficult to align and carry out when you're in pain. And if you're the caregiver, you may wonder if you can train yourself to be this sensitive when you're trying to alleviate someone's misery.

My recommendation is to concentrate on mastering the most basic communication if you're in pain and rely on a caregiver: talking about what you need right now. Instead of saying, "I'll be okay; I don't need a doctor," or "I'm too tired to see a therapist; leave me be," and instead of showing anger at a caregiver with a comment like, "You're not doing me any good!" try to connect honestly with what you need or want and reveal it. Being stoic, hiding in denial, or taking your frustration out on others cannot possibly promote healing. Such negativity creates an emotional and spiritual shutdown, which only promotes physical pain.

What do you need right now? You may mistakenly believe that it's smarter to deny your needs, to be self-protective, and to not communicate your feelings and what you're going through. If so, you may be having a real conflict between what you're willing to talk about and what you fear will hurt a relationship. This does you, and others, a real disservice.

On the other hand, if you're in pain, you may not know what to say or how to say it. Like Kate, you may be full of fears about the meaning or status of your condition, and you may try to make silence speak for you. Perhaps you need comfort and don't know how to ask for it from others. Maybe you're stir crazy and want to get out, and talking about leading a normal life makes you feel guilty. Or maybe you need more pain medication, and you worry that more drugs may become addictive or that other people will think you are weak. Or perhaps you're like many of my patients whose pain has made them re-evaluate their lives, and you want to talk to someone about how to improve things.

If you cannot talk about these issues with family or friends who are your caregivers, you have options. Write down these thoughts and feelings and make an appointment to see someone who can help you communicate your true feelings and help provide solutions. This caregiver may be a spiritual counselor, a psychotherapist, a physical therapist, your doctor, or any other health-care professional who will listen to you. Then you're on the way to real healing.

Jacques L. Bolle, a registered nurse with a PhD in counseling, is a gifted listener and a master of intuition about patients in pain. He's able to help people focus on their strengths rather than the pain, and he is always available when they want to talk. Sometimes, he told me, "people in pain feel trapped and get to a point where they feel there's no *life* in their lives. What's happened is that they've lost the critical component of aliveness along with their well-being. I try to help people move from denial and say what needs to be said. The most powerful things are for us to *be there*, to listen, and to be emotionally accessible. When you're in pain, it's not about making big changes but about making peace with what you have and knowing the value of life and laughter and what a difference they make."

Letting Others In

Caregivers can feel confused or inadequate and can even have sympathy pains. How can you make their caretaking easier for both of you? I spoke to Barbara deVries Henkind, RN, a New York public health nurse, about this topic. Her work takes her to the homes of her patients, and she sees firsthand how patients and families relate to each other. Caregivers, she stressed, don't like feeling helpless but prefer to have something to do to help relieve the pain.

"If you're taking care of someone in pain," she says, "you're taking care of the whole family. People want to help loved ones relieve their pain and are happy to have a task to do." She finds that simple tasks help families to better deal with someone who's suffering. It could be any task—giving a back massage, getting a heating pad, helping to elevate someone's leg, encouraging them to walk more, learning how to dose medication, or even buying and putting on relaxation tapes, which, in conjunction with modern medicine, can bring some relief to many people who are in pain.

Henkind says, "When family or friends have nothing to offer

or are shut out, they feel helpless or hurt. When the person in pain allows someone in, it's a bonding experience that helps everyone concerned. But you have to *want* to let others in. I had a patient with rectal cancer who was angry about having cancer and being in pain, and he couldn't get past it. Nothing his wife would do would comfort him, and his rejecting her was as hurtful as having to see him in pain. It was a hard cycle to break, because he was stuck at the anger point and couldn't move on. His wife would have done anything for him, but he wouldn't let it happen." He resisted her care and caring, determined to hold on to his suffering and unable to show his vulnerability. Meanwhile, his wife thought she had to be strong by not crying or showing her real feelings.

Dr. Bolle comments on such resistance to caregiving: "While you may want to maintain your composure and be in control of your own feelings when you care for someone, it's also healing to cry with your loved ones and be that open with each other." This is truly letting someone else in on your feelings. "It's a reflection of the society telling us we have to be productive and *do* something," he adds. "But there is a reverse script, too. Be vulnerable and understand what the other person is going through, and share the humanness." This goes both ways—from the person in pain understanding the caregiver to the caregiver understanding the person in pain.

Communicate the Details about Your Pain

When you are home, and there are family, friends, or nurses or other medical practitioners helping you, it's very helpful to keep track of the pain and what is working best to ease it. It will help your caregivers figure out what method of pain control works best for you.

Since it's important to include home-based caregivers in the development of a pain management plan, share your records with them. You may need help getting into a comfortable position, for example, and your caregiver needs to learn how to help you reposition yourself without adding any real discomfort.

If you like, you can show your caregiver the record-keeping system that I suggested in Chapter 1. Or you can start another, different record-keeping system in a little notebook that you use to record pertinent information about your pain level. I've listed 12 points related to pain that you can address in your notebook. My suggestion is for you to copy these points on the first page. Read them every day and record:

1. Words to describe your pain that day

2. Any activity that seems to be affected by the pain or that increases or decreases pain

3. Any activity that you cannot do because of the pain

4. The name and the dose of the pain medicine you are taking

5. The times you take pain medicine or use another pain-relief method

6. The number from your rating scale that describes your pain at the time you use a pain-relief measure

7. The pain rating 1 to 2 hours after using the pain-relief method

8. How long the pain medicine works

9. Pain ratings throughout the day to indicate your general comfort

10. How pain interferes with your normal activities, such as sleeping, eating, sexual activity, or working

11. Any pain-relief methods other than medicine that you use, such as rest, relaxation techniques, distraction, skin stimulation, or imagery

12. Any side effects that occur

A partial entry in your journal may look like this.

<u>August 14: Monday</u>

Woke up with headache behind the eyes and shooting back pain. Had a difficult time getting in and out of the tub, especially lifting my left leg.

Thought I might be able to put in a half day of work, but was talked out of it.

Decided to do some work at the computer, raising it on a makeshift table on the desk so I could work standing up. Sitting for more than a half hour in the same position still makes back pain worse.

Took Percocet at 8:00 a.m.

If you have any specific question or concern for a health-care professional about your condition, do not hesitate to seek an answer. The best thing you can do is to ask each person on your team what you can expect regarding pain and pain management in terms of their specialty. So, for example, if you're having acupuncture treatments or going on a new medication, ask what you can expect within a certain timeline. You may respond immediately to an acupuncture treatment, while someone else may require more time before they get the same relief. You may react to a new medication with a side effect, while someone else may have none. Report complaints of pain that is not adequately relieved, an increase in pain, a new pain or discomfort, and any side effects that develop, which may include constipation, drowsiness, and nausea.

Your caregivers need to know whether or not you're improving.

Until they find what is right for you, you may have to go through a trial-and-error period.

And a reminder: Discuss your feelings, fears, and concerns regarding pain management with your entire team. They're there for you.

Keeping Others in Touch with Your Medical Support Team

It's important for others who are helping you to have quick access to every medical professional you are seeing for your condition. You may be seeing more than one doctor or more than one specialist, so note it for others in a "Support Team Directory." This is simply a list of relevant information about each person on your medical team, with the most up-to-date contact information. You also need to list the kind of medication prescribed for you or advice given to you by each medical professional. Always include as part of this team the name of a close relative or friend who knows your condition well and can be contacted in case they are needed. If this person is at a job most of the day, include their usual work schedule and work phone number.

If you have questions that you think of for a doctor or therapist, allow yourself space to write down those questions, and include the date of your entry. If you need someone else to make a call for you, they can see who the question is for and when you asked it. So, for example, if you weren't sure if you could take your medication with food, or if you could have at least one glass of wine or beer an hour or so after taking your pills, note it next to the prescribing doctor's name, along with the date. When the question's been answered, you can check it off.

One option is to prepare this directory on a few sheets of paper stapled together and keep them near your telephone. Or, if you prefer to keep the listings on the back pages of your journal, be sure that others know where to find the information. Your directory can look like the sample on the following page.

Sample Support Team Directory

Primary doctor's name:

_____

Address:

_____

Phone:

_____

Medication(s) and dosage(s):

_____

_____

Questions or comments I have for this specialist:

_____

_____

_____

Doctor's name:

_____

Address:

_____

Phone:

_____

Medication(s) and dosage(s):

_____

_____

Questions or comments I have for this specialist:

_____

_____

_____

Nurse's name:

_____

Address:

_____

Phone:

_____

Suggested caregiving tips:

_____

_____

Questions or comments I have for this specialist:

_____

_____

_____

Pharmacist's name:

_____

Address:

_____

Phone:

_____

Prescriptions (refills and expiration dates):

_____

_____

Questions or comments I have for this specialist:

_____

_____

Social worker's name:

_____

Address:

_____

Phone:

_____

Questions or comments I have for this specialist:

_____

_____

_____

Physical therapist's name:*

_____

Address:

_____

Phone:

_____

*If your treatment plan includes more than one type of therapy, such as massage therapy and acupuncture, be sure to list the names of all the practitioners.

Type of therapy and frequency:

_____

_____

Questions or comments I have for this specialist:

_____

_____

_____

Psychotherapist's name:

_____

Address:

_____

Phone:

_____

Frequency of visits:

_____

Questions or comments I have for this specialist:

_____

_____

_____

**In Case of Emergency
Relative or friend's name:**

_____

Address:

_____

Home phone:

_____

Office phone and work hours:

_____

Comments:

_____

_____

Relating to the Caregiver

It's easy to forget that caregivers also need assurance and support. Caring for others in pain is exhausting at times. A study on the subject, called "Family Caregiver Perspectives of Pain Management," which appeared in *Cancer Practice* magazine, reported that family caregivers have become increasingly responsible for complex care and challenging pain management. Many caregiving friends and family members—some of whom are employed outside the home—often struggle "with the physical, social, psychological, and financial burdens associated with caring for a loved one in pain." Additionally, caregivers may also experience physical pain of their own as a result of the demands of caring for a patient with unrelieved pain.

Your compassion and an understanding of your caregivers' experiences can give them strength to continue helping you.

You should be aware of two very specific concerns that are common to all caregivers. By paying attention to the caregiver's feelings, you strengthen the relationship and ease their—and your—burdens.

Caregivers' Concerns about You

You may really be in pain, but your family and friends may be reluctant to acknowledge it. This is not because they don't believe you. Rather, it's because it's hard for them to face the possibility that your condition may be getting worse instead of better when, in fact, you may just be having a bad day. Furthermore, you may deny that you're in pain in order to relieve your worried caregivers.

Family caregivers also may be hindered by other fears that can become emotionally draining. They may worry about over- or undermedicating you. They may worry that you'll become "addicted" to your medications. This is why you need to include your family team in any treatment plan from its inception and put them in contact with your health-care professionals to educate them. Keeping an accurate log or journal that documents all your treatments, drugs, and doctors, like the preceding sample, will help immensely.

Genuine caregiving is more like care *sharing*. It is a partnering that develops between two people.

How Caregivers Care for Themselves

Caregivers sometimes try to do too much for the person in pain, without realizing that it's too much. At the same time, some people in pain expect caregivers to be above their feelings, to have unlimited amounts of energy and time, and to never say no to a demand. That expectation is unfair and unhealthy for both of you.

Establishing a more intimate relationship and getting closer to your caregivers involves both heart and mind. An article in *The Journal of Hospice and Palliative Care* advised caregivers that genuine caregiving involves both parties expressing emotions and establishing boundaries. There are times when it's appropriate to say no, when it makes sense for your caregiver to give herself a reprieve from the pressures she experiences. "By establishing boundaries about what you're prepared to do and what you're able to do and how much you'll be available and when and where and how and why, you can help the one you care for while you protect yourself," advise the authors of the article.

Caregivers really need to stay healthy and aware of their own needs, too. They cannot neglect their well-being. Taking time to care for themselves is not a matter of selfishness but is about staying vital so that they can be true to themselves and give you the most beneficial care. They need to sleep well, exercise, and eat wisely, as well as give themselves time off and take time away from the person they're caring for. They need to socialize, allow themselves to have fun, seek spiritual replenishment, and reinvigorate their life force.

Part of caring for themselves is being able to talk about how they feel. All caregivers want to know that their feelings matter, too, so don't hesitate to ask them how they are doing. If you ask, and they always come up with automatic responses like, "I'm okay," or "Fine, thanks," it's a clue that they're holding back. To inspire them to open up and talk, encourage a discussion with an open-ended kind of question, like those below.

- How are you doing with all of this?

- How are your spirits?

- How are you hanging in?

- Is there something I can do right now to help *you*?

- What do you need most right now?

- What's helping you get through this?

- What's going through your mind as you try to cope with all of this?

- Are there any obstacles to your coping?

Most of all, stay connected, show gratitude to those who care about you, and heal!

Sharing Optimism and Keeping Up Hope

I spoke with James Avery, MD, senior medical director of the Visiting Nurse Service of New York Hospice Care, the largest hospice in America. Dr. Avery works with people who have very little time left and who are looking for a final sense of peace. Although hospice patients may have to give up hope for a cure, and thus, for more life, there are other hopes to reach for. "What I found is people feel like rusted cars in a junkyard—they don't feel lovable and tend to push people away. But hope can be redefined and refocused," says Dr. Avery. "What I do is give patients homework. It is for them to give love and say it and show it to their families, and to accept love in return. This becomes a turning point, a profound renewal."

Being able to connect with others in love is as true for people in final hospice care as it is for you—pain sufferers who have a lot of life ahead of you. I urge you not to give in to pain but to fight it. Embrace life and start the joy now. I encourage you to reach for pain management solutions, to welcome in caregivers, to sustain meaning in your life, to build a spiritual foundation, and to know you are loved.

CHAPTER 9

Heal Your Pain

Creating a Treatment Plan
That Works for You

If there are any two big truths about pain, they are that healing cannot be done alone and that healing is not the same for everyone. Every chronic pain sufferer needs the guidance and support of a unique and sympathetic team, whose size will vary according to individual needs.

I deal with migraines and a chronic back problem of my own on a regular basis. I know what kind of support I need to remain as highly functioning as possible. I could not exist without a spiritual connection to a higher being and an equally powerful connection to my family. My work, helping others relieve their pain, also provides another meaning to my life. I take sumatriptan (Imitrex) for migraines and see an acupuncturist to relieve backaches.

How would you describe your situation? How do you need to heal yourself?

There's hardly anyone with pain who needs *only* medical management. You've read all the stories so far and have learned a wide spectrum of ways to help yourself and be helped. When you know what kind of specialist to see and what you need to encourage healing, you can devise a treatment plan. With a plan, you can:

- Become an active partner in your health care so that pain no longer limits your chances for living a full and happy life.

- Be willing to try new techniques for pain control.

- Seek assistance when you need it.

- Learn to detach from the past and look ahead with a measure of optimism.

- Confront any issues that cause mood change or depression.

- Give yourself permission to ask for what you want and not play the victim.

- Know that you're doing everything possible to heal yourself.

Here are my suggestions for putting together the most effective plan for yourself. It begins with your willingness to deal with any emotional issues that still weigh heavily in your life, and with letting them go.

Be True to Yourself

Negative feelings have no value. Be willing to lose them or defuse them! You have the courage to work on any areas in your life that add to your pain. Since your pain may not only be caused by a physiological condition, please take this opportunity to examine how you feel. Go back to the sections in this book that deal with anger, depression, stress, having a purpose in life, spiritual connections, and forgiveness, and think about how you would assess your psychological state regarding these factors. Are you still angry or depressed over events of the past that you cannot change? Do those events add to your real physical pain now?

If you need to see a spiritual counselor, a social worker, a nurse, or a psychotherapist, do yourself a favor and add this person to your team. What matters is that you are able to open up to this person about your problems and that you are listened to. Seek a counselor interested in treating people with chronic illnesses who will know how to deal with your pain.

Work with a Doctor Who Is Right for You

You don't have to go to a pain management specialist to find the doctor who is right for you and who can treat your pain effectively. Other practitioners may be family doctors, internists, or any other primary care doctors who can manage your case and special needs. Your choice of doctor may also depend on where you live and your community.

How do you know which doctor is right for you?

Most doctors are vitally connected to the needs of their patients. We know that we cannot make an accurate diagnosis unless we listen to the patient. We are aware of the advances in our particular fields and apply them when it is possible or necessary. My personal philosophy is simple: Every patient is an individual and must be treated individually. At the same time, I hope my patients understand what is wrong with them, what they can do to help heal themselves, and what I must do to make them feel better. The best indication of whether a doctor is right for you is if you can say yes to the following questions after discussing your case.

Is my doctor a partner in my health care? This is *the* critical question to ask yourself. Do you feel as if your doctor cares about you and is interested in your case? Or do you get the distinct impression that the doctor expects you to do as he suggests without question, including accepting options for drug therapy or surgery?

Part of this partnership is the doctor's willingness to go beyond traditional medicine if you are interested in trying a complementary modality for your condition. A lot of pain relief involves trial and error—especially with complementary therapies. Can you benefit from massage therapy, for example, or could Reiki make a difference in your comfort level? Doctors cannot know exactly what will work with every patient, so sometimes it is a matter of "trying it on" and seeing what therapy will work.

Your best bet is to find a doctor who will be there with you through your healing journey and can manipulate the system to provide what you need. Helen's story shows clearly what I mean.

I met Helen after a speech I gave at a large hospital. She'd driven from her Baltimore home to hear my talk, with the idea of seeing me professionally. Helen, an operating room nurse, had been through 2 remarkable years, going from perfectly healthy to having pain as a constant companion. She decided to seek my advice about her pain management program and told me the course of events that had changed her life so dramatically.

A few years earlier, Helen had elective surgery to remove a bunion on her right foot. It's a perfectly common operation, but 3 months later, Helen's foot wasn't healing. Her primary care doctor assured her that some people heal faster than others and that she shouldn't worry. Then, while playing with her 4-year-old daughter, she fell off a porch and fractured the baby toe on her left foot. Now, she said, "both feet were a mess. The foot that had been operated on hurt all the time, and I couldn't walk on it." This accident sent her to a large hospital, where she told her doctor that she wasn't healing and feared she had some serious problem.

Her doctor told her to use a wheelchair and stay off her feet so they could take a look at what was underlying the problem. She was not allowed to drive, and walking caused her serious pain. Helen's doctor started her on the painkiller Percocet. She told me she was "blown away" that at age 42 she couldn't walk, and she was frustrated with the pain. The doctor suggested the need for a bone biopsy, not an easy procedure, and not one that Helen wanted to do. Finally, her doctor convinced her it would be worth the effort. Her tests showed that she had osteopenia (a condition that precedes osteoporosis) *and* osteoporosis. It meant that her bones weren't able to heal properly.

At her doctor's recommendation, Helen started on an experimental injectable drug that was not approved by the FDA. The drug is supposed to stimulate bone production, which she was lacking. Slowly but surely, her bones started to heal. Finally, she found relief, and even better, she could walk without painkillers. However, as a side effect of the experimental drug, she had some back pain.

When Helen went off the experimental drug, her doctor put her on alendronate (Fosamax), a drug that treats osteoporosis. This doctor also suggested she try acupuncture treatments for her back.

"There are so many therapies, and I'll try them one at a time while I still live with some discomfort," Helen said. She then asked me, "Am I on the right track?"

After hearing her story, it sounded to me as if her doctors were understanding, on top of the newest therapies, and were helping her. I could hear in this story that Helen and her primary care doctor had the right kind of rapport that would best help solve her pain problems.

Since I believe that acupuncture treatments help many but not all people, I thought it was worth her time to find out if she would benefit from them. Before we parted, Helen said, "I'm actually grateful that I had that elective bunionectomy and then fell off the porch! I'm grateful that I had a doctor I believed in and who listened to me. I'm happy just to take a walk with my husband and kids."

Can I talk about my medical problems with my doctor? Do you feel comfortable enough with your doctor that you are not intimidated into silence, thereby omitting essential information about your pain? Does your doctor listen to you and understand what you are saying? If you can't speak freely with your doctor, you are doing yourself a disservice. Find another doctor with whom you have the right chemistry.

Do I feel confidence in my doctor's ability? You must feel that your doctor understands your condition and that he is willing to explain it to you. Can he correctly diagnose and treat your problem so that it doesn't get worse over time? If you're seeing a doctor who keeps telling you that you need to learn to live with pain, then he may be either missing the diagnosis or not treating you appropriately. If you feel flagging confidence in your doctor, remember that you are entitled to a second or third opinion. Don't worry what the first doctor will think if he finds out. It is your body, your health, and your right to seek the best medical care to heal your pain!

Believe You Can Heal

Managing pain isn't easy at any point, but you will come out healed if you commit yourself to a treatment plan that tackles all of your issues. Take it one step at a time and never waver in believing you can do more for yourself.

You have an opportunity to leave a positive legacy despite the burden of pain. Stay connected to the world. Believe in yourself and in self-respect. Show gratitude for life, be generous with yourself and others, and keep your sense of humor.

You can only come out of the pain experience with a greater joy for life and compassion for others.

appendix

In this appendix, I've included extra copies of the charts and logs provided earlier in the book. Use these extras to track your pain and your treatment plan beyond the initial 2 weeks.

Pain Management Logs

1. Tracking Your Pain Level Day by Day

In the chart on page 200, make a check mark in the box that corresponds with the day of the week and your specific pain level. For example, if it is Tuesday, and you had moderate to more severe neck pain, you might enter a check mark in the Tuesday column corresponding to number 6 or 7.

At the end of each day, answer the questions in Step 2, providing specific information about the pain you did or didn't feel that day.

2. Describing Your Pain Day by Day

Write down what did or didn't happen to you because of the pain. You can use the Daily Pain Description Log on page 202. Provide as much information as possible about your pain level by answering these questions.

- How many times did you feel pain? It could be none, once, 10 times—however many times it happened.

DAILY PAIN LEVEL LOG

FIRST WEEK

Pain	Mon.	Tues.	Wed.	Thur.	Fri.	Sat.	Sun.
10							
9							
8							
7							
6							
5							
4							
3							
2							
1							
0							

- List where you felt pain. Was it, for example, in your neck, back, wrists, abdominal area, or all over your body?

- Did any specific activity start the pain? If so, which activity? Were you, for example, climbing stairs, lifting a child, or doing chores such as laundry, vacuuming, and so on?

- How did the pain interfere with your normal activities, such as sleeping, eating, sexual activity, or working efficiently?

- Every day, note if you avoided, limited, or canceled any activity or social engagement because of pain or changes in how

Weeks of _____

SECOND WEEK							
Pain	**Mon.**	**Tues.**	**Wed.**	**Thur.**	**Fri.**	**Sat.**	**Sun.**
10							
9							
8							
7							
6							
5							
4							
3							
2							
1							
0							

you felt, including working at your job. What changes did you make?

• Did you call your health-care professional between visits because of pain?

So, for example, your entry for Tuesday might read:
"Felt sharp, pulling pain four times in neck. Pain started up driving to work, getting caught in traffic jam, and having to keep turning my head. Slight slowdown at work until late afternoon because of intense, stiffening neck pain and pounding headache. Canceled dinner with my in-laws."

(continued on page 206)

FIRST WEEK

MONDAY	
TUESDAY	
WEDNESDAY	
THURSDAY	
FRIDAY	
SATURDAY	
SUNDAY	

	SECOND WEEK
MONDAY	
TUESDAY	
WEDNESDAY	
THURSDAY	
FRIDAY	
SATURDAY	
SUNDAY	

MEDICATION AND TREATMENT LOG

FIRST WEEK

MONDAY	
TUESDAY	
WEDNESDAY	
THURSDAY	
FRIDAY	
SATURDAY	
SUNDAY	

Healing Pain

SECOND WEEK

MONDAY	
TUESDAY	
WEDNESDAY	
THURSDAY	
FRIDAY	
SATURDAY	
SUNDAY	

3. Medications, Treatments, and Therapies

The chart on page 204 will help you track how medications, treatments, and therapies do or do not affect your pain. There are six simple questions, and they should take you only a minute or two to answer.

- What is the name of the medication? Did you take it according to your doctor's instructions?

- Did you skip a dose? If so, why?

- Did the medication help relieve your pain?

- Did you still have breakthrough pain even though you took the medication?

Duplicate Logs

DAILY PAIN LEVEL LOG							
FIRST WEEK							
Pain	Mon.	Tues.	Wed.	Thur.	Fri.	Sat.	Sun.
10							
9							
8							
7							
6							
5							
4							
3							
2							
1							
0							

- Did you have any side effects after taking the medication? Typical side effects include lack of appetite, drowsiness or sleepiness, nausea, vomiting, upset stomach, or constipation.

- Did you do anything to help relieve your pain other than take prescription medication?

For example, on Wednesday, you might say:
"Neck pain woke me up last night so took two aspirin. This morning, pain felt like it was pulling or sharp; took a Percocet to relieve it. Felt better for 4 hours. Headache developed late afternoon, but was bearable. Took another Percocet and felt better. After work, took hot bath, massaged neck."

Weeks of _____

SECOND WEEK							
Pain	Mon.	Tues.	Wed.	Thur.	Fri.	Sat.	Sun.
10							
9							
8							
7							
6							
5							
4							
3							
2							
1							
0							

DAILY PAIN LEVEL LOG

FIRST WEEK

Pain	Mon.	Tues.	Wed.	Thur.	Fri.	Sat.	Sun.
10							
9							
8							
7							
6							
5							
4							
3							
2							
1							
0							

Weeks of _____

SECOND WEEK Pain	Mon.	Tues.	Wed.	Thur.	Fri.	Sat.	Sun.
10							
9							
8							
7							
6							
5							
4							
3							
2							
1							
0							

DAILY PAIN DESCRIPTION LOG

FIRST WEEK

MONDAY	
TUESDAY	
WEDNESDAY	
THURSDAY	
FRIDAY	
SATURDAY	
SUNDAY	

Healing Pain

SECOND WEEK

MONDAY	
TUESDAY	
WEDNESDAY	
THURSDAY	
FRIDAY	
SATURDAY	
SUNDAY	

DAILY PAIN DESCRIPTION LOG

FIRST WEEK

MONDAY	
TUESDAY	
WEDNESDAY	
THURSDAY	
FRIDAY	
SATURDAY	
SUNDAY	

Healing Pain

SECOND WEEK

MONDAY	
TUESDAY	
WEDNESDAY	
THURSDAY	
FRIDAY	
SATURDAY	
SUNDAY	

MEDICATION AND TREATMENT LOG

FIRST WEEK

MONDAY	
TUESDAY	
WEDNESDAY	
THURSDAY	
FRIDAY	
SATURDAY	
SUNDAY	

SECOND WEEK

MONDAY	
TUESDAY	
WEDNESDAY	
THURSDAY	
FRIDAY	
SATURDAY	
SUNDAY	

MEDICATION AND TREATMENT LOG

FIRST WEEK

MONDAY	
TUESDAY	
WEDNESDAY	
THURSDAY	
FRIDAY	
SATURDAY	
SUNDAY	

SECOND WEEK

MONDAY

TUESDAY

WEDNESDAY

THURSDAY

FRIDAY

SATURDAY

SUNDAY

Building a Team: Where to Find Medical Professionals

I've provided a list of contacts for a range of specialists so you can find one in your area. Speak to your primary doctor before starting any complementary modality and consider any limitations you may have.

Pain Management

American Academy of Pain Medicine
4700 West Lake Avenue
Glenview, IL 60025
Phone: 847-375-4731
www.painmed.org

American Chronic Pain Association
PO Box 850
Rocklin, CA 95677-0850
Phone: 800-533-3231
www.theacpa.org

American Pain Foundation
201 North Charles Street, Suite 710
Baltimore, MD 21201-4111
Phone: 888-615-PAIN (7246)
www.painfoundation.org

American Pain Society
4700 West Lake Avenue
Glenview, IL 60025
Phone: 847-375-4715
Fax: 877-734-8758
www.ampainsoc.org

International Association for the Study of Pain
909 NE 43rd Street, Suite 306
Seattle, WA 98105-6020
Phone: 206-547-6409
www.iasp-pain.org

Acupuncture

National Certification Commission for Acupuncture and Oriental Medicine
11 Canal Center Plaza, Suite 300
Alexandria, VA 22314
Phone: 703-548-9004
Fax: 703-548-9079
www.nccaom.org

Biofeedback

Biofeedback Certification Institute of America
10200 West 44th Avenue, Suite 310
Wheat Ridge, CO 80033
Phone: 303-420-2902
Fax: 303-422-8894
www.bcia.org

Complementary and Alternative Medicine

National Center for Complementary and Alternative Medicine
National Institutes of Health
NCCAM Clearinghouse
PO Box 7923
Gaithersburg, MD 20898
Phone: 888-644-6226
TTY/TDY: 866-464-3615
Fax: 866-464-3616
http://nccam.nih.gov

Guided Imagery

Academy for Guided Imagery
30765 Pacific Coast Highway, Suite 369
Malibu, CA 90265
Phone: 800-726-2070
Fax: 800-727-2070
www.academyforguidedimagery.com

Hospice and Palliative Medicine

American Academy of Hospice and Palliative Medicine
4700 West Lake Avenue
Glenview, IL 60025
Phone: 847-375-4712
Fax: 877-734-8671
www.aahpm.org

American Hospice Foundation
2120 L Street NW, Suite 200
Washington, DC 20037
Phone: 202-223-0204
www.americanhospice.org

Hypnosis

American Council of Hypnotist Examiners
700 South Central Avenue
Glendale, CA 91204
Phone: 818-242-1159
Fax: 818-247-9379
www.hypnotistexaminers.org

National Board for Certified Clinical Hypnotherapists
1110 Fidler Lane, Suite 1218
Silver Spring, MD 20910
Phone: 800-449-8144 or 301-608-0123
Fax: 301-588-9535
www.natboard.com

Massage Therapy

American Massage Therapy Association
500 Davis Street, Suite 900
Evanston, IL 60201-4695
Phone: 877-905-2700 or 847-864-0123
Fax: 847-864-1178
www.amtamassage.org

National Certification Board for Therapeutic Massage
and Bodywork
1901 South Meyers Road, Suite 240
Oakbrook Terrace, IL 60181
Phone: 800-296-0664 or 630-627-8000
Fax: 630-214-3902
www.ncbtmb.com

Reiki
International Association of Reiki Professionals
PO Box 6182
Nashua, NH 03063-6182
Phone: 603-881-8838
www.iarp.org

Spiritual Ministry and Counseling
Your best bet for locating a practitioner in spiritual counseling is
to contact a large local hospital in your area and ask if they have
someone on staff who does this therapy. You can also inquire if
that person has taken the appropriate courses in clinical pastoral
education.

Yoga
American Yoga Association
PO Box 19986
Sarasota, FL 34276
Phone: 941-927-4977
www.americanyogaassociation.org

references

Ambuel, Bruce, Waukesha Family Practice Center, Waukesha, WI. "Taking a Spiritual History #19." *Journal of Palliative Medicine* 6, no. 6 (Nov. 2003): 932.

"Animal Attraction." Bonus section, *Time*, Nov. 2003.

"Back Pain." *Newsweek*, Apr. 26, 2004, 44–48.

Brady, Marianne J., Amy Peterman, et al. "A Case for Including Spirituality in Quality of Life Measurement in Oncology." *Psycho-Oncology* 8, no. 5 (1999): 417–28.

Bruera, Eduardo, and Hak Nam Kim. "Cancer Pain." *Journal of the American Medical Association* 290 (Nov. 12, 2003): 2476–79.

Charlish, Anne, and Angela Robertshaw. *Secrets of Reiki*. Woodland Hills, CA: *Natural Health* Magazine/DK Publishing Inc., 2001.

Chochinov, Harvey Max. "Thinking Outside the Box: Depression, Hope, and Meaning at the End of Life." *Journal of Palliative Medicine* 6, no. 6 (Nov. 2003): 973–75.

DeAngelis, Catherine D. "Pain Management." *Journal of the American Medical Association* 290 (Nov. 12, 2003): 2480–81.

Frank, Arthur W., edited by Jonathan E. Dostrovsky, et al. "How Stories Remake What Pain Unmakes." In *Proceedings of the 10th World Congress on Pain, Progress in Pain Research and Management*. Seattle: IASP Press, 2003.

Frankl, Viktor E. *Man's Search for Meaning*. New York: Simon and Schuster, 1963.

Handel, Daniel, and Sarah Handel. "Nonpharmacologic Management of Cancer Pain." In *Advances in Cancer Pain: A Bedside Approach*. Manhasset, NY: CMP Healthcare Media/Oncology Publishing Group, 2005.

Kane, Javier. *Spirituality in Medicine*. Department of Pediatrics/Division of Hematology, Oncology, Immunology, and Palliative Medicine Fellowship Program, Christus Santa Rosa Hospice, San Antonio, Texas, 2000.

Kass, Jared D. "Contributions of Religious Experience to Psychological and Physical Well-Being: Research Evidence and an Explanatory Model." *The Caregiver Journal* 8, no. 4 (1991): 199–205.

Kass, Jared D., and Lynn Kass. *Manual/Resources for Resilience: Building a Resilient World View through Spirituality*. Cambridge, MA: Behavioral Health Education Initiative, Greenhouse, Inc., 2000.

Kirkhart, Beverly. *My Healing Companion*. Santa Barbara, CA: Comeback Press, 2001.

Lesho, Emil. "When the Spirit Hurts: An Approach to the Suffering Patient." *Archives of Internal Medicine* 163 (Nov. 10, 2003): 2429–30.

Management of Cancer Pain. Clinical Practice Guideline, Number 9. U.S. Department of Health and Human Services, 1994.

Mannes, Andrew, Russell R. Lonser, et al. "Interventional Neurosurgical Approaches for Treating Severe Pain." In *Advances in Cancer Pain: A Bedside Approach*. Manhasset, NY: CMP Healthcare Media/Oncology Publishing Group, 2005.

Mäntyselkä, P. T., E. A. Kumpusalo, et al. "Chronic Pain and Poor Self-Rated Health." *Journal of the American Medical Association* 290 (Nov. 12, 2003): 2435, 2438–39.

Margoles, Michael, and Richard Weiner, eds. *Chronic Pain: Assessment, Diagnosis and Management*. Boca Raton, FL: CRC Press, 1999.

Mazanec, Polly, and Judy Bartel. "Family Caregiver Perspectives of Pain Management." *Cancer Practice*, May/June 2002: S66–S68.

McBride, LeBron J., Gary Arthur, et al. "The Relationship between a Patient's Spirituality and Health Experiences." *Family Medicine*, Feb. 1998: 122–26.

"Medical Advances." *USA Weekend*, Mar. 5–7, 2004: 8, 10.

Meldrum, Marcia L. "A Capsule History of Pain Management." *Journal of the American Medical Association* 290 (Nov. 12, 2003): 2470–71.

Miller, James E. "The Grit and Grace of Being a Caregiver." *American Journal of Hospice and Palliative Care*, May/June 1995: 18–21.

Otis-Green, Shirley, Rhonda Sherman, et al. "An Integrated Psychosocial-Spiritual Model for Cancer Pain Management." *Cancer Practice*, May/June 2002: S58–S65.

Pain Control. National Institutes of Health/National Cancer Institute, June 2000.

Pain Notebook. The American Pain Foundation.

Pain Report: An Update on Issues, Research, and Treatment Trends. Dannemiller Memorial Educational Foundation, Sept. 2003: 3–4.

Penson, Richard T., Rushdia Z. Yusuf, et al. "Losing God." *The Oncologist* 6, no. 3 (2001): 294–95.

Pereira, Donna L., and Diane C. St. Germain. "Pharmacologic Adjuvant Therapy for Cancer Pain." In *Advances in Cancer Pain: A Bedside Approach*. Manhasset, NY: CMP Healthcare Media/Oncology Publishing Group, 2005.

Principles of Analgesic Use in the Treatment of Acute Pain and Cancer Pain. 3rd ed. American Pain Society, 1992.

"Prolonging the Agony." *Science*, July 16, 2004: 326–29.

"Questions and Answers about Using Magnets to Treat Pain." *NCCAM (National Center for Complementary and Alternate Medicine) Newsletter*, Fall 2004: 3.

Starlanyl, Devin, and Mary Ellen Copeland. *Fibromyalgia and Chronic Myofascial Pain Syndrome: A Survival Manual*. Oakland, CA: New Harbinger Publications, 1996.

Stewart, W. F., Richard Lipton, et al. "Lost Productive Time and Cost Due to Common Pain Conditions in the U.S. Workforce." *Journal of the American Medical Association* 290 (Nov. 12, 2003): 2443–44.

"Taking a New Look at Pain." *Newsweek*, May 19, 2003: 44–46.

"The Pain Truth." *Good Housekeeping*, May 2003: 83–84.

"Who'll Stop the Pain." *Modern Maturity*, July/Aug. 2002: 64.

Zalaquett, Carlos P., and Richard J. Wood, eds. *Evaluating Stress: A Book of Resources*. Vol. 2. London: Scarecrow Press, 1998.

index

Assessment of pain. *See*
    Self-assessment of pain
Attitude, positive, importance of, 59,
    63, 64, 83

B

Back pain, 5–6, 155
Bayer, 144
Biofeedback, 165, 219
Biofeedback Certification Institute of
    America, 219
Boundaries, caregiver-patient, 189
Breakthrough pain, 13, 148–49
Breathing problems, as side effect of
    drugs, 153
Breathing techniques
    for stress reduction, 18–19
    in yoga, 168
Bufferin, 144
Burdens
    questions for analyzing, 125–29
    releasing
        by forgiving self and others,
            132–33
        by grieving losses, 61–62,
            131–32
        for healing, 118
        by seeking help, 61–62, 129–30
    understanding, 123–25

C

Cancer pain
    others' tolerance of, 70
    spirituality and, 112
    story about, 140–41, 144
Carbamazepine, 151
Caregivers
    communication with, 175
        about details of pain, 180–83
        elements of, 89–90, 177–79

    lack of, 175–77
    openness to, 179–80
    questions for, 190
    concerns of, about patient, 189
    needs and problems of, 188, 190
    relationship with, 174
    role of, 175
    self-care for, 189–90
    sharing medical support team
        information with, 183–88
Celebrex, 146
Celecoxib, 146
Change, 63, 83, 133
Chronic pain
    beginning healing process for, 53
    causes of, 13
    characteristics of, 12–13, 44
    coping styles for, 44–45
    depression with, 13, 46, 53
    effects of, 43–44, 45
    endorphins and, 8, 10
    incidence of, 5, 9
    opiates for, 139–40
    psychological effects of, 45, 46
    psychological questions about,
        46–47
        on attitude toward healing,
            59–65
        on real vs. imagined pain, 47–53
        on reasons for depression,
            53–57
        on reasons for stress, 57–59
    seeking medical help for, 147
    stress and, 57
    types and mechanisms of pain
        with, 13–14
    undertreatment of, 9
Codeine, 149
Communication
    with caregivers
        about details of pain, 180–83
        elements of, 89–90, 177–79

lack of, 175–77
openness to, 179–80
questions for, 190
in doctor-patient relationship,
49–50
about pain, 15–17, _15_
Complementary therapies
benefits of, 158, 159–60
candidates for, 158
consulting doctor about,
172–73
definition of, 158
doctors' openness to, 194
finding practitioners of, 173,
219–21
history of, 160
popularity of, 159–60
reasons for choosing, 161–62,
172
types of, _162_
acupuncture, 163–64
arts therapies, 166–68
biofeedback, 165
guided imagery, 164
hypnosis, 164–65
magnets, 171–72
massage, 169
meditation, 165–66
Reiki, 170–71
yoga, 168–69
"Confidence in Life and Self"
questionnaire, 104
Confusion
about pain, stress from, 54, 84
as side effect of drugs, 154
Constipation, as side effect of drugs,
154
Contracts, for opiate use, 143–44
Control, regaining, for achieving
optimism, 138
Coping style, questions about,
74–78

Counseling
refusal of, 129–30
seeking, 130, 193–94, 221
Cryosurgery, 155

D

Daily Pain Description Log, 33,
38–39, 202–3
duplicates of, **210–13**
how to use, 36, 199–201
Daily Pain Level Log, 33, **34–35,**
200–201
duplicates of, **206–9**
how to use, 35, 199
Darvocet, 150
Darvon, 149–50
Daypro, 145
Definition of pain, 6, 8
Demerol, 150
Denial of pain, 5
Depression
with chronic pain, 13, 46,
53
help for, 54, 56–57, 86–87
reasons for, 53–54
analyzing, 54–56
Descriptions of pain
logs for (_see_ Daily Pain
Description Log; Daily Pain
Level Log)
questions analyzing, 20–21
words for, _15_
Desipramine, 151
Dilaudid, 149
Disbelief of pain
by medical professionals and
others, 15–17, 46, 47–49,
51–52, 53
reasons for, 50–51
Distraction, for managing pain,
137–38

M

Magnet therapy, 161, 171–72
Massage, 169, 220–21
Meaning of life, finding, 119
Medical professionals. *See also*
    Doctors
    effect of loss on, 82
    where to find, 218–21
Medical support team directory
    how to use, 183
    sample, 184–88
Medical view of spirituality, 111–13
Medication and Treatment Log, 33,
    40–41, 204–5
    duplicates of, **214–17**
    how to use, 36–37, 206–7
Medications. *See* Drug therapies
Meditation, 165–66
Meloxicam, 146
Men, pain in, 9, 10, 11, 50
Meperidine, 150
Methadone, 141, 144, 149, 150
Migraines
    chronic vs. recurring, 13
    medications for, 145
Mobic, 146
Morphine, 147, 149, 150
Music therapy, 167–68
Myofascial pain, 14

N

Naproxen, 144, 145
National Board for Certified Clinical
    Hypnotherapists, 220
National Center for Complementary
    and Alternative Medicine,
    219
National Certification Board for
    Therapeutic Massage and
    Bodywork, 221

National Certification Commission
    for Acupuncture and Oriental
    Medicine, 219
Nausea and vomiting, as side effect
    of drugs, 153, 154
Negative emotions and thoughts
    defusing, 193–94
    with depression, 87
    effects of, 59, 64, 111
Nerve damage, pain sensations and,
    7
Nerve destruction, neuropathic pain
    from, 14
Neuromas, cryosurgery for, 155
Neuropathic (nerve) pain, 14, 150,
    151
Neurosurgical techniques, 154–56
Nicotine addiction, 143
Nociceptors, pain sensations and, 7,
    14
Nonmalignant pain, incidence of, 5
Nonsteroidal anti-inflammatory
    drugs (NSAIDs), 14, 144–46,
    146, 148
Nontraditional therapies. *See*
    Complementary therapies
Norpramin, 151
NSAIDs. *See* Nonsteroidal anti-
    inflammatory drugs

O

Opiates
    addiction to, 143
    adjuvants and, 151
    contracts for use of, 143–44
    definition of, 148
    effectiveness of, 147–48
    physical dependence on, 141–42,
        143
    psychological dependence on,
        142–43

Relationships
  bad, exacerbating pain, 84–85
  caregiver-patient (*see* Caregivers)
  effect of pain on, 66–70
  importance of, 70–71, 81–83
  questions about, 24–26, 71–74
  steps for improving, 85–86
    being honest about needs, 89–90
    being honest about pain, 87–89
    dealing with depression, 86–87
    giving up rescue fantasies, 86
    journaling, 91
    resisting isolation, 90–91
Religion, vs. spirituality, 99, 100–103
Rescue fantasies, as obstacle to
    healing, 86
Respiratory depression, as side effect
    of drugs, 153
Rofecoxib, 146

S

Salt glow, 160
Sedation, as side effect of drugs, 153
Self-approval, importance of, 83
Self-assessment of pain
  how to begin, 19–20
  importance of, 17–18, 53
  logs for (*see* Daily Pain Description
    Log; Daily Pain Level Log)
  questionnaire for, 20–33
Self-esteem, importance of, 83–84
Senses, required for healing, 64–65
Sequential trials, 157
Side effects of drugs, managing, 151,
    153–54
Sleep deprivation, from pain, 153
Sleepiness, as side effect of drugs,
    153
Somatic pain, 14, 145
Spinal-fusion surgery, 6
Spiritual advisors, 104, 221

Spiritual assessment questionnaires
  purpose of, 101–2, 103–4
  sample, 31–33, 105–10
Spirituality
  affecting quality of life, 102
  author's view of, 113–17
  importance of, 97–98
  keys to using, 117–19
  loss of, 99–100
  meaning of, 98–99
  medical view of, 111–13
  optimism from, 102–3
  vs. religion, 99
  religious view of, 100–103
  sources of, 96–97, 98–99
  stories of, 95–97
Statistics on pain, 9
Strengths, for reclaiming self,
    137–38
Stress
  from anger, 133
  breathing affected by, 18–19
  from confusion about pain, 84
  effects of, 57–58
  loss of spirituality from, 99–100
  from negative relationships, 68
  pain and, 10, 57, 58
  physical symptoms of, 57
  productive, 58
Stress reduction
  methods of, 59
    breathing technique, 19
    journaling, 91
    from pain management, 33
Stress-related disorders, 57
Suffering
  addressing, in holistic healing, 113
  definition of, 8
  effects of focusing on, 97
  methods of relieving, 8
  sources of, 111
Support groups, 90, 129–30

about the authors

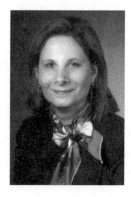 Ann Berger, MSN, MD, is one of the foremost specialists in pain management in the nation. A medical oncologist specializing in pain treatment, she has written and edited numerous books on pain and palliative care for patients and health-care providers. Dr. Berger is also senior editor of the most widely used textbook on palliative care, *Principles and Practice of Palliative Care and Supportive Oncology*. She currently resides in Darnestown, Maryland.

C. B. deSwaan is a New York City–based freelance writer specializing in nonfiction. She has written 20 books with expert collaborators, including the best-selling *Men Are Just Desserts* and *Smart Cookies Don't Crumble*.